W9-CNL-287

GIFTED HANDS

More Praise for *Gifted Hands*

"I have been especially delighted to have the opportunity to read Dr. Schwartz's splendid book. I have enjoyed not only his encyclopedic overview of American surgery but also his lucid writing on this fascinating subject, to which he himself has made important contributions as a teacher and an innovator."

—Harold Ellis, PhD, CBE, FRCS, emeritus professor of surgery, University of London, and author of *Cambridge Illustrated History of Surgery*

"Seymour Schwartz has given us a remarkably researched account of the rise of surgery in America. Through the gripping storytelling of one of the country's master knife wielders, a splendidly readable account of surgeons and their craft is now on hand. This book delivers it all and more. From the stirring description of early nineteenth-century studies in gastric physiology, to the dramatic narrative of twenty-first-century heart transplants, Schwartz uses his lifetime's experience in the vineyard of surgery to relate this most fascinating of medical tales. Magisterial in its scope, Gifted Hands *honors the nation's surgeons and their deeds as few books have done before."*

—Ira Rutkow, MD, former clinical associate professor of surgery, University of Medicine and Dentistry of New Jersey, and author of *American Surgery: An Illustrated History*

"From the frontier heroism and scientific dedication of McDowell and Beaumont, to the cascade of achievements in cardiac and transplantation surgery, and the advanced technology of today, Gifted Hands *is an inspiring journey led by a uniquely authoritative guide. Concise yet rich in detail, Schwartz's book provides a superb distillation of the rise of American surgery to its present position of preeminence."*

—Daniel R. Roses, MD, Jules Leonard Whitehill Professor of Surgery and Oncology, New York University School of Medicine

"This gripping account of the leaps that put surgery in the vanguard of the healing arts and life sciences reflects the philosophy of John Stuart Mill that all social changes are products of the actions of extraordinary individuals. Schwartz, himself one of the world's preeminent surgeons and medical scholars, has identified individuals who changed surgery and the barriers they broke down, from antiquity to recent times. What a great read for everyone!!!"

—Thomas E. Starzl, MD, PhD, professor of surgery, University of Pittsburgh

GIFTED HANDS

America's Most Significant Contributions to Surgery

SEYMOUR I. SCHWARTZ, MD

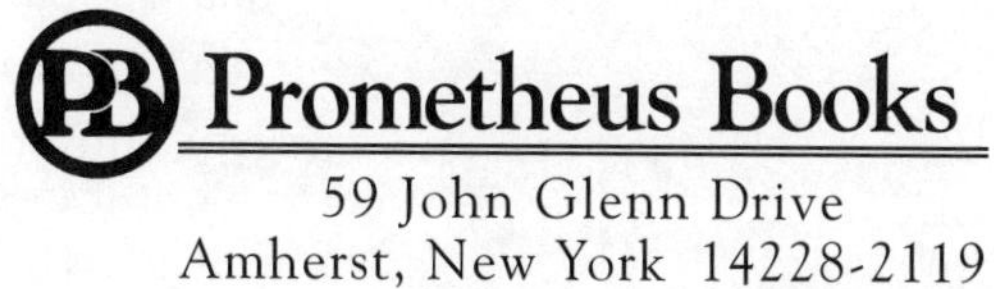

59 John Glenn Drive
Amherst, New York 14228-2119

Published 2009 by Prometheus Books

Inquiries should be addressed to
Prometheus Books
59 John Glenn Drive
Amherst, New York 14228–2119
VOICE: 716–691–0133, ext. 210
FAX: 716–691–0137
WWW.PROMETHEUSBOOKS.COM

13 12 11 10 09 5 4 3 2 1

Library of Congress Cataloging-in-Publication Data

Schwartz, Seymour I., 1928–.
Gifted hands : America's most significant contributions to surgery / Seymour I. Schwartz.
p. cm.
Includes bibliographical references and index.
ISBN 978–1–59102–683–9 (hardcover : alk. paper)
1. [DNLM: 1. Surgery—history—United States. 2. History, Early Modern 1451–1600—United States. 3. History, Modern 1601—United States. 4. Surgical Procedures, Operative—United States. WO 11 AA1 S399g 2009].

RD27.3.U6S39 2009 2004
617.0973—dc22 2008046815

Printed in the United States on acid-free paper

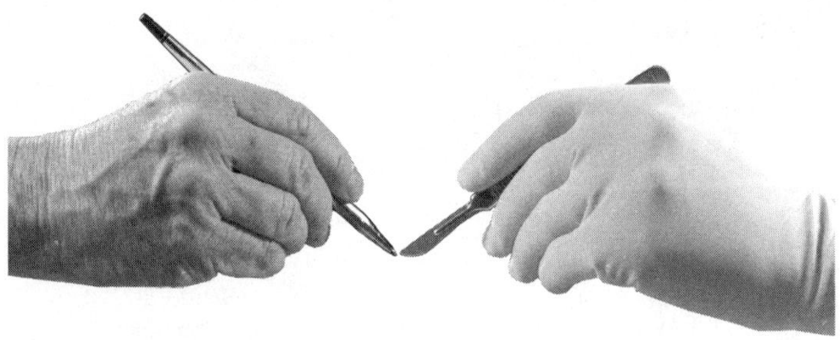

The deeds of surgery, represented by the scalpel, comprise the art that separates a disease from a patient, repairs a defect, stems the effects of trauma, and reconstructs the anatomy to achieve normalcy or functionality.

The words of surgery, represented by the pen, describe the technical accomplishments and scientific advances.

The technical accomplishments and scientific advances of the past have created a contemporary cornucopia of surgical therapy. Progress in the past and present times form the evident bases for anticipation of an even more exciting future.

—Seymour I. Schwartz, 2008

CONTENTS

Dedication

To all the surgeons who have crossed my path and particularly those of the profession whose presence and productivity have enriched my surgical life.

PREFACE

Surgery undoubtedly is superior to medicine for the following reasons:

1. *Surgery cures more complicated maladies, such as toward which medicine is helpless.*

2. *Surgery cures diseases that cannot be cured by any other means, not by themselves, not by nature, nor by medicine. Medicine indeed never cures a disease so evidently that one can say that the cure is due to medicine.*

3. *The doings of surgery are visible and manifest while those of medicine are hidden, which is very fortunate for many physicians.*

—*Treatise on Surgery*
Henri de Mondeville (1260–1320)

In the latter half of the nineteenth century, Theodor Billroth, a German professor working in Vienna and the world's preeminent surgeon, proclaimed with an eye to the future: "It was the goal of our time to make out of surgical art a science."[1] Now, as the twenty-first century is coursing through its first decade, that goal has been achieved. The science of surgery that has evolved from the art of surgery is, largely, an achievement of the twentieth century, and one dominated by American surgeons. As a consequence, the United States currently enjoys an essentially unchallenged role of leadership in the field of surgery.

Prior to the twentieth century's explosive growth in the science of surgery on American soil, there were several primitive contributions that took place in the new nation, as well as an occasional major or seminal advance. The surgical contributions that occurred in North America during the first three centuries that followed the initial European settlement of the continent (the 1600s through the 1800s) lacked the complexity of more modern work and were mainly isolated events. As such, they lend themselves to a chronological consideration. By contrast, the contributions that evolved during the twentieth century are complex, often incorporating several interdependent achievements. Therefore, they are best considered in specialty categories.

At a time when the United States existed for a mere twenty-six years, it was an American surgeon who initiated the entire practice of abdominal surgery that would spread throughout the world. A quarter of a century later, it was another American surgeon who opened the road to the science of surgery by conducting the first deliberate physiologic studies on a human being. In the first half of the nineteenth century, the surgical correction of pathologic disorders in women was advanced by an American surgeon. Before that century had reached its midpoint, America offered the world of surgery its greatest boon by making an operative procedure painless through the development of inhalation anesthesia.

In the second half of the nineteenth century, two of the most common disorders that demanded surgical attention, gallbladder disease and appendicitis, had surgical approaches initiated by American surgeons and physicians. Before the nineteenth century came to an end, an American surgeon created a filing and retrieval system that continues to this day to facilitate the accumulation and acquisition of medical information. Another American surgeon developed a model for training surgeons that, with some modification, is also used to the present day.

During the twentieth century, surgery underwent exponential growth and America proved to be the most fertile breeding ground for advances in the science throughout the entire world. The diverse fields of vascular surgery, cardiothoracic surgery, transplantation, and the maintenance of homeostasis (physiological equilibrium) throughout all aspects of surgical care have benefited from initiatives made by American surgeons.

As a consequence of past and recent contributions, American surgery has earned a leadership role within the discipline. The path from European disregard and even disdain for American surgeons has been a short one in the history of medical science. This short journey, however, has been particularly fascinating and encompasses dramatic scenarios, intriguing personalities, improbable associations, and individuals of heroic proportion.

This book is aimed at both interested lay readers and members of the medical profession. For the former, explanations of the medical terms have been provided to facilitate a deeper technical understanding of the science. For my medical colleagues, I appreciate your patience with this, as we all explore together the fascinating and innovative history of surgery in America.

ACKNOWLEDGMENTS

The genesis of this work can be dated to the preparation for the video "America's Contributions to Surgery" that was prepared for distribution by Roche to surgeons in 1992. I am indebted to James T. Adams, Irwin Frank, and Marshall Lichtman, three medical colleagues who over the years have added valuable suggestions after reviewing this manuscript, just as they have for many of my previous works. This also applies to Melinda Beard. C. Rollins Hanlon contributed significantly when, in response to providing a review for the dust jacket, he offered extensive and most appropriate editorial corrections. Gianna Nixon-Saldinger provided invaluable assistance in the preparation of the illustrations. Linda Regan, who has edited two of my recent books, added significantly, and John Silbersack has continued to offer guidance through the world of publishing.

CHAPTER 1:

PRE-COLUMBIAN AND COLONIAL TIMES

All hold this Tantram [surgery] to be the most important of all the other branches of Áyurveda [science of medicine], in as much as instantaneous actions can be produced. . . . It is eternal and a source of infinite piety, imparts fame and opens the gates of Heaven to its votaries, prolongs the durations of human existence on earth, and helps men in successfully fulfilling their missions, and earning a decent competence in life.

—Sushruta-Samhitá (fifth century BCE)
"Sutrasthánam"

The term "surgery" came to the English language from the French word "chirurgien," which in turn derives from the Latin (and ultimately Greek) words "cheir," meaning the hand, and "ergon," meaning work. Thus, the art and the science of surgery focus on manual activities that contribute to patient care. It can hardly be regarded as a modern discipline, and surgery can claim priority as the subject matter of the oldest extant scientific document, *The Edwin Smith Papyrus.* This extraordinary dissertation, dating from the seventeenth century BCE, is a copy of a manuscript that was written during the age of the Pyramids, circa 3000 BCE. The document, which some have attributed to Imhotep, reports forty-seven instances of trauma; each is addressed in a consistent and logical sequence of examination, diagnosis, and treatment. The papyrus includes reference to the cranial sutures, the brain, spinal fluid, comminuted and compound fractures, and the use of cautery.[1] The forty-eighth case (case number 46 in the document) makes a probable reference to cancer of the breast in a man. The Egyptians certainly had a sophisticated medical culture.

The Native Americans on the northern continent of the New World, before their exposure to European sophistication, had their own approach to surgical problems. The early reports of English and European explorers and settlers provide brief glimpses of Native American incursions in the realm of surgery. John Smith, who played a leadership role in the establishment of the first permanent English settlement at Jamestown, Virginia, wrote in *A Briefe and True Report of the New Found Land of Virginia*: "For swellings also they use smal peeces of touchwood, in the forme of cloves, which pricking on the griefe, they burne close to the flesh, and from thence draw the corruption with their mouth. With this root *wighsacan* they ordinarily heal green wounds; but to scarifie a swelling or make an incision, their best instruments are some splinted stone. Old ulcers or putrified hurtes are seldome seen cured amongst them."[2]

One of the most common forms of minor surgical procedures was scarification of the skin that was resorted to for "almost all Distempers." The instruments employed included rattlesnake fangs from which the venom had been removed and sharp pieces of obsidian and flint.[3] Scarification was also used as a counterirritant in patients with persistent pain. In 1714 John Lawson, described how Native Americans amputated the feet of their captives and grafted skin over the exposed end.[4] Along similar lines, in the latter half of the eighteenth century, it was reported that the Ojibwas, near Lake Nipigon, repaired accidentally torn ears: "They cut them smooth with a knife and sew the parts together with a needle and deer's sinews."[5] To do this, North American Indians used sutures of human hair, deer tendons, and vegetable fibers, especially basswood, while South American Indians used leaf-cutting ants as clips, twisting off their heads after they approximated cut ends of skin.[6]

Mark Catesby, the English artist-naturalist who provided the Europeans with the first description of the fauna and flora of Carolina, Florida, and the Bahamas, wrote in 1754: "Indians are wholly ignorant in Anatomy, and their Knowledge in surgery is very superficial; amputation & phlebotomy they are strangers to; . . . the cures of ulcers and dangerous wounds is facilitated by severe abstinence, which they endure with a resolution and patience peculiar to themselves."[7] The Potawotamis cleansed wounds with a syringe made of a quill and an animal bladder.[8] The most complex procedure performed during the pre-Columbian period was trephination, which placed burr holes through the skull in order to remove evil spirits. Instruments used for this procedure in Peru by the early Incas have been uncovered, and there is additional evidence that the North American Indians performed trephination as well.

Over two centuries before these reports concerning Native American surgical procedures were published in the eighteenth century, the first chronicled operation performed in North America appeared in print. The operation, which was but a small segment of a major saga, brings into focus a riddle: How did the head of a cow impact on the history of American surgery? The simple answer is that Alvar Nuñez Cabeza de Vaca, whose name is translated, "head of a cow," was responsible for the 1542 publication of a detailed description of his removal of an arrowhead from the sternal region of a Native American in the southwestern part of the country about 1535.

The name Cabeza de Vaca was taken by the explorer from his mother, Teresa Cabeza de Vaca, who was a descendant of a thirteenth-century Spanish shepherd named Martin Alhaja. During the Christians' reconquest of Spain from the Moors, Alhaja marked a mountain pass with the skull of a cow, thereby facilitating a surprise attack by King Sancho of Navarre at the battle of Las Navas de Tolosa in 1212. As a consequence, the Spanish king bestowed upon the shepherd the title of "Cabeza de Vaca," which was perpetuated with pride by the maternal side of the hero's family.

In 1527, the explorer Cabeza de Vaca left Spain as the treasurer and second in command to Panfilo de Narvaez, who planned to take possession of the Gulf Coast from Florida to the Rio de las Palmas. The expedition eventually landed on the shore of present-day Tampa Bay in April 1528. Narvaez took off with the main body of men on an exploration and was never seen again. Cabeza de Vaca, with the remaining 247 troops, constructed boats and attempted to reach the northernmost part of eastern Mexico. A storm wrecked most of the boats, and Cabeza de Vaca and a few survivors reached the shore of either Galveston Island or nearby San Luis Island early in November of the same year.

From 1528 to 1534, all those who had reached land died, with the exception of Cabeza de Vaca and three of his companions, who, from 1528 to 1536, lived among the natives and eventually trekked overland to Culiacán on the west coast of Mexico and then on to Mexico City before returning to Spain in 1537. In the latter half of 1535, either in southwestern Texas or northern Mexico, Cabeza de Vaca removed an arrowhead from an Indian's chest. The procedure is detailed in Cabeza de Vaca's *La Relación* (1542), which was first published in Zamora, Spain, with a second edition published in Valladolid, Spain, in 1555. Only two copies of the first edition are extant, one in the Biblioteca de España in Madrid and the other in the New York Public Library. A translation of the description of the operation reads:

> Here they brought a man to me whom they said had been wounded by an arrow a long time before, in the right side of his back. They said that the arrowhead was lodged over his heart. He said that it hurt a great deal and that it caused him to suffer all the time. I touched him and felt the arrowhead and noticed that it had gone through cartilage. With a knife that I had, I opened his chest through to that spot, and saw that the arrowhead had gone through and would be very difficult to remove. I cut further, stuck the point of the knife in, and at last removed it with great difficulty. It was very long. With a deer bone, I practiced my trade as a physician and gave him two stitches. After I had stitched, he was losing a lot of blood. I stopped the bleeding with hair scraped from an animal skin. When I removed the arrowhead they asked me for it and I gave it to them. The entire village came to see it and they sent it further inland so that the people there could see it. Because of this cure they made many dances and festivities, as is their custom. The following day I cut the stitches and the Indian was healed. The incision I had made looked only like one of the lines in the palm of one's hand, and he said that he felt no pain or suffering at all. And this cure gave us such standing throughout the land that they esteemed and valued us to their utmost capacity.[9]

The operative report is an early example of surgical hubris: the surgeon admired his own stitching and the resulting imperceptible scar. During the fiftieth anniversary celebration of the Texas Surgical Society in 1965, Dr. Robert Sparkman of Dallas commissioned Tom Lea to paint a representation of the operation. The original hangs in the Library of the University of Texas Medical Branch in Galveston (fig. 1).

The first operation that was performed on a colonist found its way into print in Increase Mather's *Remarkable Providences Illustrative of the Earlier Days of American Colonization* (1684), the year before he became president of Harvard College. A child was struck by the undercarriage of a cart between her right ear and the crown of her head. The skull was pierced and brain tissue extruded through the wound. Some of the soft matter was pressed back into the wound and a dressing was applied. A silver plate was kept in place over the dressing for a while to protect the wound. The child lived to become the mother of two children and did not demonstrate any mental deficit.[10]

The first two published accounts of elective surgical procedures in the colonies are both credited to Zabdiel Boylston, the Boston physician for whom a street in that city is named as a consequence of his championing

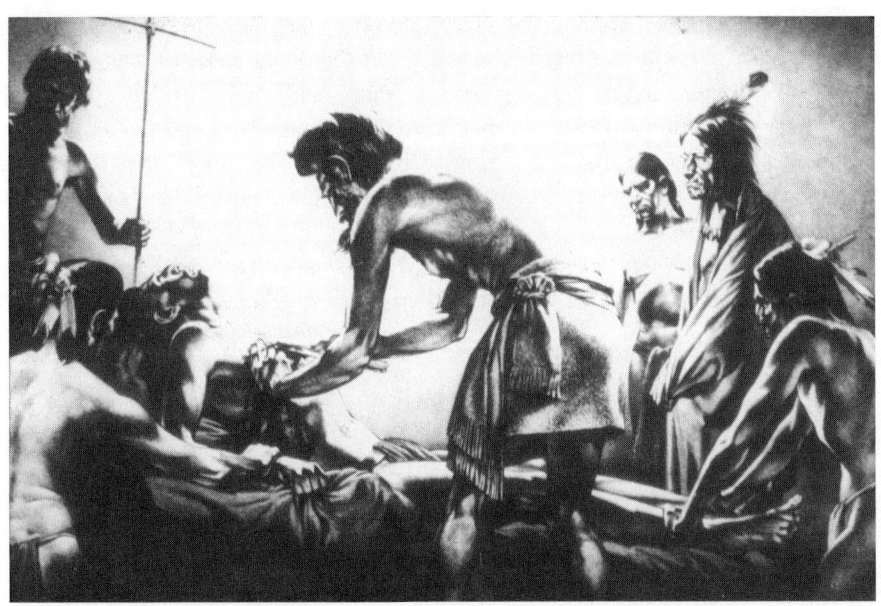

Figure 1: Thomas Lea painting that depicts Cabeza de Vaca's removal of an arrowhead from the chest of an Indian. Courtesy of Blocker History of Medicine Collections, Moody Medical Library, University of Texas Medical Branch, Galveston, Texas.

smallpox inoculation. In the Boston *News-Letter* for the week of July 17, 1710, a successful cutting for bladder stone was reported:

> Henry Hill Distiller in the town of Boston New-England, having had a Child grievously afflicted with the Stone, apply'd himself to Mr. Zabdiel Boylston of the said Boston, Practioner in Physick and Chirurgery; who on the 14th of June last, in the presence of sundry Gentlemen, Physicians and Chyruriens, Cut the said Child & took out of his bladder a stone of considerable bigness, and with blessing of God in less than a months time has perfectly cured him, and hold his water. This is the third Operation on the Stone on Males and Females, and all with good success. He Likewise pretends to all other operations in Surgery, Which Operations the said Hill could not omit to make Public.

Boylston's next reported operation, the removal of a cancerous breast, was reported in the *Boston Gazette* for the week of November 21, 1720.

> For the Public Good of any that have or may have Cancers, These may Certify. That my wife had been laboring under the dreadful Distemper of a Cancer of the Left Breast for Several Years, and altho' the Cure was attempted by Sundry Doctors from time to time, to no effect; And when Life was almost despair'd of by reason of its repeated bleedings, growth & stench, and there seemed immediate hazard of Life, we send for Doctor Zabdiel Boylston of Boston, who on the 28th of July 1718 in the presence of several Ministers & others assembled on that occasion cut her whole Breast off; and by the Blessing of God on his Endeavors, she has obtained a perfect Cure. I deferred the Publication of this, lest it should have broke out again.
>
> —Edward Winslow
> Rochester, October 14, 1720[11]

The most notable surgeon in colonial America was unquestionably John Jones, who was born in Jamaica, New York, in 1759, and died in Philadelphia at the age of sixty-two (fig. 2). Initially trained by his father and cousin in Philadelphia, John Jones studied abroad with William Hunter, Colin MacKenzie, and Percival Pott at St. Bartholomew's Hospital in London. John Jones continued his studies in Paris and received a doctorate in medicine from the University of Rheims in 1751. His reputation was established at the battle of Lake George in 1755 during the French and Indian War, at which time he treated the French general Baron Diskau, who had been captured by the victorious William Johnson. Johnson, in spite of his appellation of "White Savage," consequent to his acceptance by the Iroquois, protected the wounded prisoner and allowed him to recover and return home.

In 1767, Jones was among a small group of distinguished physicians who petitioned for a medical section at King's College, now Columbia University. He became the first professor of surgery in the colonies in what is regarded to be the second-oldest colonial medical school, antedated by two years by the College of Philadelphia, later the University of Pennsylvania. His *Introductory Lecture to His Course in Surgery* (1767) anticipated the credo of modern academic surgeons:

> Surgery may, with great propriety, be divided into medical & manual. The first comprehends an infinite variety of diseases which require the assistance of both internal and external applications; the last is confin'd to those cases which admit of relief from the hand alone, or assisted with instru-

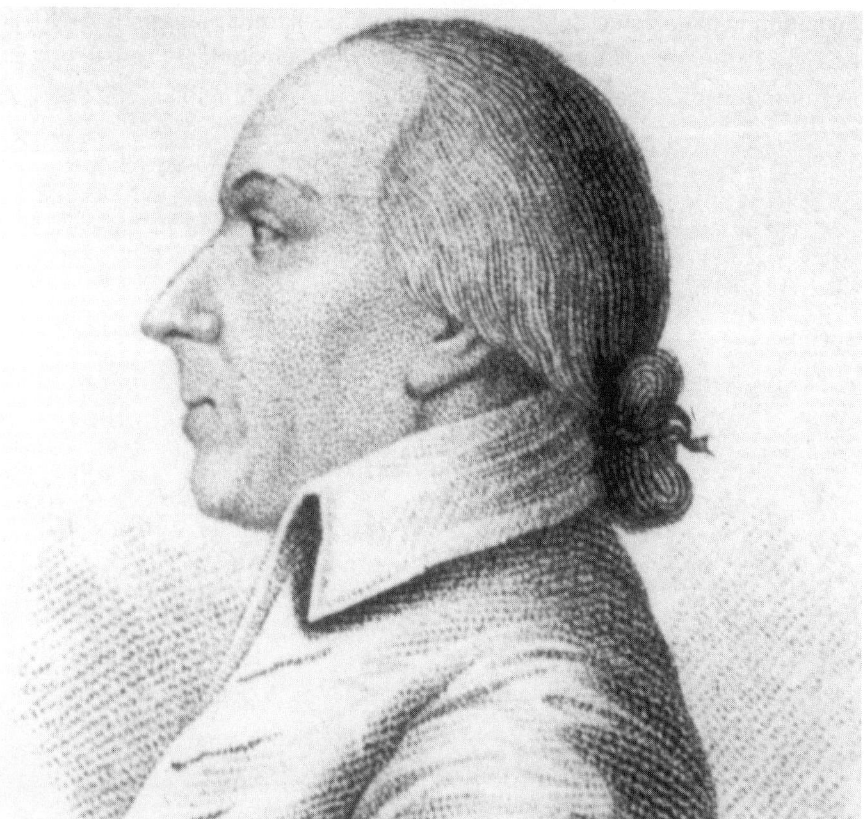

Figure 2: John Jones. Courtesy of Edward G. Miner Library, University of Rochester School of Medicine and Dentistry, Rochester, New York.

> ments. . . . An operation alone is but a single point in the curve of diseases; a knowledge of the causes which require it, the accidents which attend it, & the treatment which may vary, according to the variety of these accidents are the most essential objects in the art of surgery.[12]

Jones later participated in the formation of the New York Hospital. At the onset of the military activities during the American Revolution, Jones produced the first medical text printed in the colonies, *Plain, Concise, Practical Remarks on the Treatment of Wounds and Fractures: To Which Is Added a Short Appendix on Camp and Military Hospitals; Principally Designed for the Use of Young Military Surgeons in North America* (1775), which served as a manual for military surgeons engaged in caring for the troops. Jones's reputation is manifested in his call to care for Benjamin Franklin in 1790, at the time of Franklin's terminal illness. Shortly thereafter, he assisted at an operation for treatment of a carbuncle on George Washington.

CHAPTER 2:

THE PROFESSOR AND THE PIONEER

The public, who are so ready to determine on the merits of our profession, and even the patients whoare to suffer, are surprisingly ignorant both of the Surgeon's motives for what he does, and the propriety of the methods he puts in practice. He is continually operating in secret as a matter of necessity. The most sensible give the decision up to him; so that he is answerable to his own conscience, and to that alone.

—*Illustrations of the Great Operations in Surgery*
Sir Charles Bell (1774–1842)

The victory achieved by the thirteen colonies that ended the American Revolution was formalized by the Treaty of Paris in 1783, which established the boundaries of a new and independent nation. The independence was mainly political, since commercial and intellectual relationships retained many elements of the previous interdependence with Great Britain. Americans continued to call on Great Britain and Europe for intellectual sophistication and guidance in the sciences, including surgery. A significant identity for American surgery would not be established until the end of the nineteenth century. Before that time, however, there were occasional bursts of brilliance.

During the first decade of the nineteenth century, as a new nation was gradually developing its standing in the world, two disparate surgeons helped raise the curtain on the American surgical scene. One was a distinguished professor who conducted his practice in the most urban and highly populated city in the United States, whereas the other was a relatively unknown surgical pioneer, operating in a small frontier community. It was the latter who dramatically revolutionized the entire field of abdominal surgery throughout the world. Although the two never met, their intellectual paths crossed in a telling circumstance.

The professor, Philip Syng Physick (1768–1837) (fig. 3), was born into a distinguished Philadelphia family; his father was the Receiver General of Pennsylvania and the Keeper of the Great Seal. After graduating from the University of Pennsylvania, Philip Syng Physick studied under the noted English surgeon John Hunter, who offered Physick a position as his assistant. Instead of accepting the flattering invitation, Physick proceeded to the University of Edinburgh, where he received a doctorate of medicine in 1792 before returning to establish a practice in the city of his birth. Benjamin Rush, a signer of the Declaration of Independence and America's most notable physician of the time, was among his referring medical colleagues.

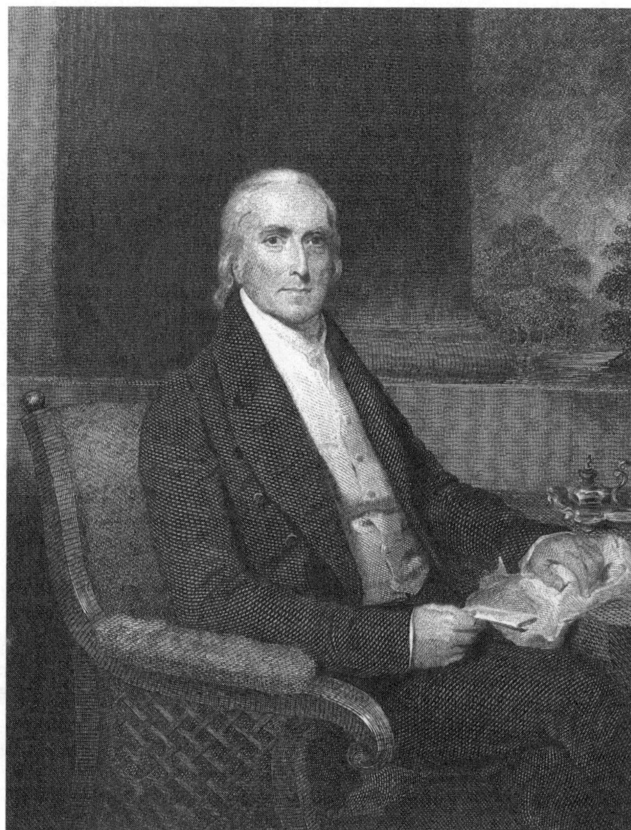

Figure 3: Philip Syng Physick. Courtesy of Edward G. Miner Library, University of Rochester School of Medicine and Dentistry, Rochester, New York.

In 1794, Physick was appointed surgeon to the Pennsylvania Hospital, a position that he held until 1816. The Pennsylvania Hospital was the first hospital to be built within the thirteen colonies. The cornerstone was laid in 1754, in large part due to the efforts of Dr. Thomas Bond and Benjamin Franklin. The Pennsylvania Hospital was preceded in the Western Hemisphere by only three institutions. In 1524, the Hospital de Jesús opened its doors in Mexico and remains in continuous use. In 1639, Hôtel-Dieu was established in Quebec, and five years later, a hospital with the same name had its inception in Montreal.

Physick was elected the first president of the Philadelphia Academy of Medicine and also served as professor of surgery at the University of Pennsylvania from 1805 to 1819. He contributed minimally to the medical literature, but he is credited with two significant advances. Although tubes had been inserted through the mouth into the stomach since antiquity, Physick was the first to report the insertion of a gastric tube through the mouth into which an emetic was instilled and poisonous material evacuated from the stomach, thereby saving the life of the patient. This probably evolved from John Hunter's use of a tube constructed of eel skin to feed a patient who was unable to swallow.[1] Physick also was the first to describe the use of absorbable sutures that he had made of buckskin, fox skin, and catgut to approximate disrupted tissues.

He had a large clinical practice, and he operated in the oldest extant operating room in the United States at the Pennsylvania Hospital. This room was unique in design in that it was built adjacent to a recovery room; this setup eventually developed into a pattern that remains in current hospitals. On December 27, 1805, Physick operated on a man and removed a seven-pound tumor from his parotid (salivary) gland. The specimen is preserved in the museum of the Pennsylvania Hospital. But Physick's most notable operation was the removal of over one thousand stones from the urinary bladder of John Marshall, who was then the seventy-four-year-old chief justice of the United States. A large silver serving bowl, given by Justice Marshall to his surgeon as an expression of appreciation, remains on display at the Physick House in Philadelphia.

Physick's academic position, clinical prestige, and original contributions all played a part in his appellation of the Father of American Surgery" He was described as a grave, melancholic, unfriendly, and socially insular man. His "high forehead, aquiline nose, thin and compressed lips, a finely formed mouth, and hazel eyes with their searching and, at times, penetrating gaze" reflected his personality, and his complexion was "one of extreme paleness."[2] He was "of medium height and slight build, [and] was meticulous in his dress. He was seldom seen without his powdered wig, and never abandoned the outmoded queue, a braid of hair. He had passed his life in a certain diurnal movement and rotation, any deviation of which put him to inconvenience."[3]

Physick, the distinguished and lionized surgical leader, played a minor, tangential role in the drama acted out by a pioneering surgeon in a small and distant Kentucky community west of the Allegheny Mountains. The drama that forever changed the world of surgery took place in the small city of Danville in Kentucky, which had entered the Union as the fifteenth state in 1792. Danville was established in 1781 and served as the state's first capital for a brief period of time. In 1809, at the time that surgery witnessed the first major American advancement, the city had somewhere between three hundred and one thousand inhabitants.

The pioneering surgeon Ephraim McDowell (1771–1830) (fig. 4), was born in Rockbridge County, Virginia, but moved with his family to Danville when he was thirteen years old. He had undergone a preceptorship in medicine with Doctor Alexander Humphreys of Staunton, Virginia, for two or three years before becoming a student at the University of Edinburgh in 1793. His presence in Edinburgh did not coincide with that of Philip Syng Physick, who left about six months before McDowell arrived. McDowell remained at Edinburgh for two years but did not acquire a medical degree. During that period, he elected to become a pupil of John Bell, who taught anatomy and surgery outside the confines of the university and also wrote the biography of Physick for Samuel D. Gross's *Lives of Eminent Physicians and Surgeons of the Nineteenth Century* (1861).

McDowell, the first surgeon to establish a practice west of the Allegheny Mountains, returned to Danville in 1795, where, according to a letter that he received while at Edinburgh: "Indians are still very troublesome on the frontiers from North to South."[4] Shortly after his return, he developed an extensive surgical practice that drew patients from hundreds of miles in what was then referred to as the Southwest. Although the rural surgeon had no national recognition, he was well regarded locally and was the busiest practitioner west of the Allegheny Mountains. As testimony to an impressive practice and an equally impressive surgeon, up to the year 1828, according to Samuel D.

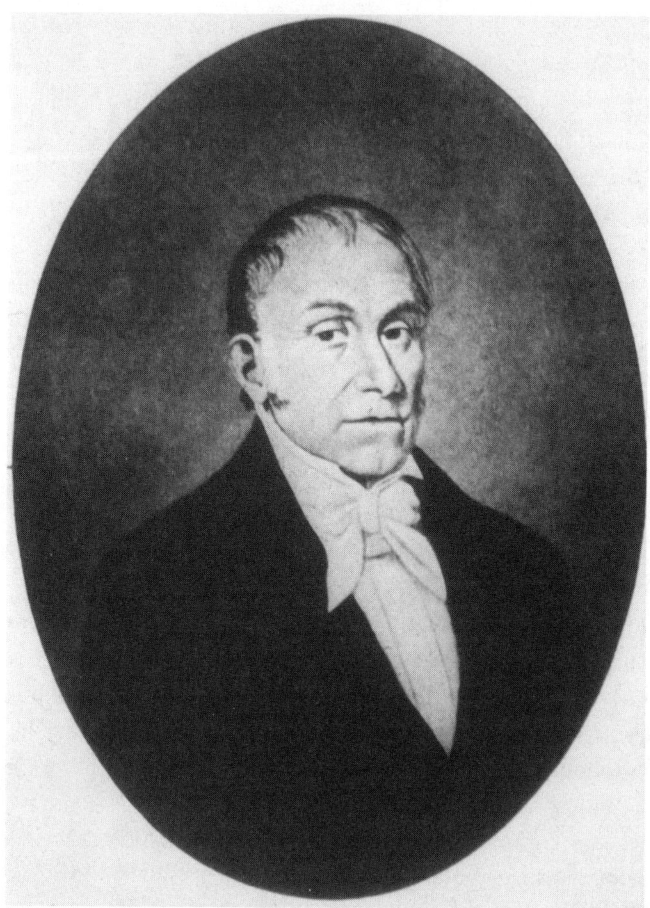

Figure 4: Ephraim McDowell. Courtesy of McDowell House, Danville, Kentucky.

Gross, McDowell had performed thirty-two lithotomies (the removal of bladder stones) without the loss of a single life.[5]

McDowell has been described as nearly six feet in height, "inclined to corpulency with a florid complexion and intense black eyes."[6] He was witty with a keen sense of humor. A deep interest and kindness characterized his care of patients, and he was noted for his retiring disposition, modesty, and generosity to his colleagues.

In spite of his acquired reputation, McDowell never became a member of the faculty of a medical school. It is particularly surprising that he was overlooked by Transylvania University, which had its origin as the Transylvania Seminary in Danville in 1785 before it moved and became the Transylvania University at Lexington, and, as such, the first notable school of higher education west of the Allegheny Mountains. During his lifetime, he was recognized for his accomplishment on only two occasions. In 1817, the year that his experience with removal of the ovary was first published, the Medical Society of Philadelphia honored him; and in 1825, the University of Maryland bestowed upon him an honorary degree, doubtless due to the influence of Dr. John Beale Davidge, one of the university's founders and a personal friend of McDowell.

Little emphasis has been accorded to the obvious fact that, throughout the ages, the dramatic episodes in surgery involved at least two indispensable participants: a daring surgeon, who is usually the recipient of recognition, if not adulation, as a consequence of the achievement; and a courageous patient, who rarely is accorded justifiable praise. In the case of the surgical breakthrough, consisting of the first chronicled successful removal of the ovary and, also, the first successful elective operation within the peritoneal cavity, the surgeon, Ephraim McDowell, displayed boldness, and the patient, Jane Todd Crawford (fig. 5), demonstrated extraordinary courage.

Mrs. Crawford died unrecognized by society at age seventy-eight in 1842, outliving her surgeon. The initial expression of an appreciation of her role did not come until 1879 when, in Danville, at the unveiling of a monument honoring Ephraim McDowell, Dr. Lewis A. Sayre, president of the American Medical Association, paid the patient a tribute:

> Another fact strokes me very forcibly, Mr. President, and that is, the heroic character of the woman who permitted this experimental operation to be performed upon her. The women of Kentucky in that period of her early history were heroic and courageous, accustomed to brave the dangers of the tomahawk and scalping-knife, and had more self-reliance and true heroism than is generally found in the more refined society of city life; and hence the courage. Mrs. Crawford, who, conscious that death was inevitable from the disease with which she suffered, so soon as this village doctor explained to her his plan of affording her relief, and convinced her judgment that it was feasible, immediately replied, "Doctor, I am ready for the operation; please proceed at once and perform it." All honor to Mrs. Crawford! Let her name and that of Ephraim McDowell pass down in history together as the founders of ovariotomy! [7]

Hero met heroine on December 13, 1809, near Greensburg, Kentucky, about sixty miles from Danville. Initially, Mrs. Crawford had been thought to be pregnant, but when it became apparent to her local physician that not pregnancy but a large abdominal tumor was the cause of her condition, McDowell was called to her home to make a diagnosis and suggest treatment. McDowell recalled the meeting in his 1817 published report:

> Having never seen so large a substance extracted nor heard of an attempt or success attending any operations such as this required, I gave to this unhappy woman information of her dangerous situation. She appeared willing to undergo the experiment, which I promised to perform if she would come to Danville.[8]

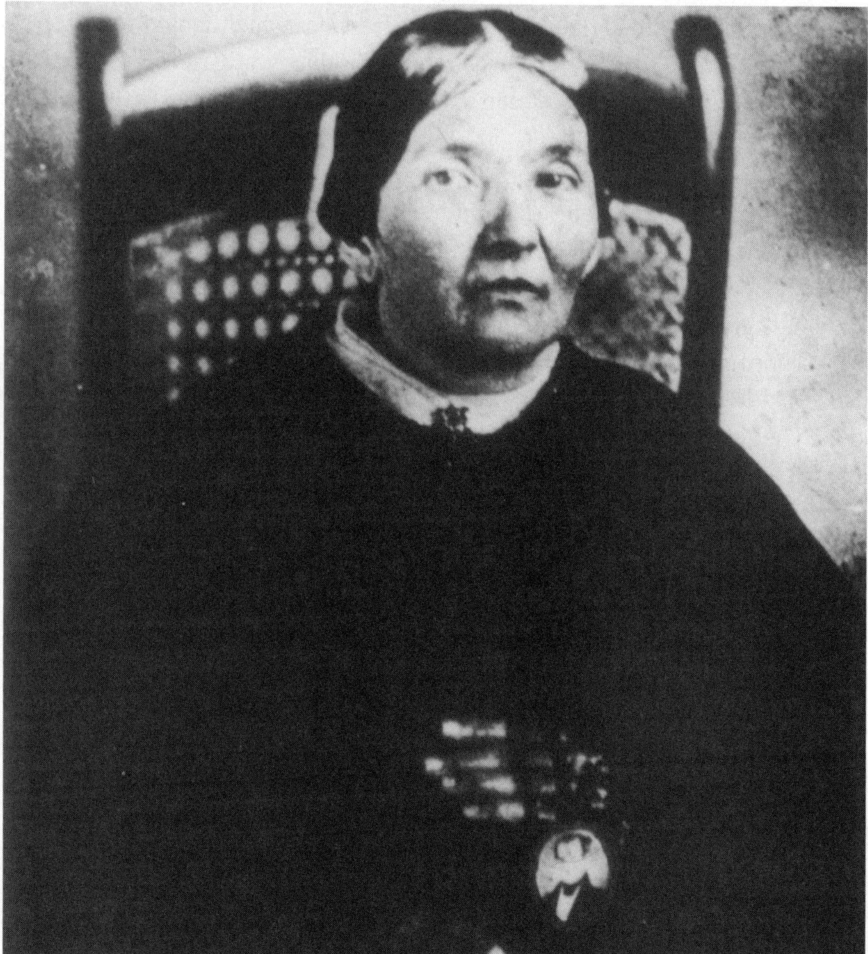

Figure 5: Jane Todd Crawford. Note that she is displaying a medallion portrait of Ephraim McDowell. Courtesy of McDowell House, Danville, Kentucky.

The intrepid patient wasted no time and made the journey alone on horseback over several days, resting the massive tumor on the horn of the saddle. The operation was performed on Monday, Christmas Day 1809. The selection of an unusual time for a surgical procedure was in keeping with McDowell's policy to operate, usually, on Sundays because the citizenry was engaged in religious and family affairs and less likely to be curious about what the surgeon was doing.

McDowell performed the operation with the assistance of Dr. James McDowell, a nephew and partner, who attempted to persuade his uncle not to operate. The procedure probably took place in McDowell's home, perhaps in an upstairs bedroom, certainly without anesthesia, which would not become available for more than three decades. It is said that Mrs. Crawford distracted herself during the procedure that lasted twenty-five minutes by repeating psalms.

Professor George Kasson Knapp painted a portrait of Ephraim McDowell and a depiction of the momentous operation (fig. 6) based solely on his artistic imagination. The painting was shown at a meeting of the American Medical Association and, over the years, has been offered inappropriately as a graphic chronicle of the event.

According to McDowell's description as it appears in his publications, the left side of the abdomen was opened with a nine-inch longitudinal incision. The left Fallopian tube was ligated, a cystic ovarian mass was opened, and fifteen pounds of gelatinous material was removed. The remaining seven and a half pounds of solid tumor were excised, the abdominal cavity was drained of blood, and the incision was closed. In five days, the patient was ambulating and making up her bed. In twenty-five days, she returned home alone on horseback.

The timing of the report of the momentous operation is indicative of McDowell's personality. He was self-effacing and sought no publicity. He purposefully delayed submission of the report of his achievement for eight years until he had replicated his success two more times. This is in sharp contrast to action of another trailblazing surgeon, Theodor Billroth. In 1881, Billroth, at the time professor of surgery at the University of Vienna and unquestionably the world's most influential surgeon, on the occasion of performing the first successful partial gastrectomy, arranged for the case report to appear in a journal six days after the event took place.

After McDowell successfully partially removed an ovarian tumor or

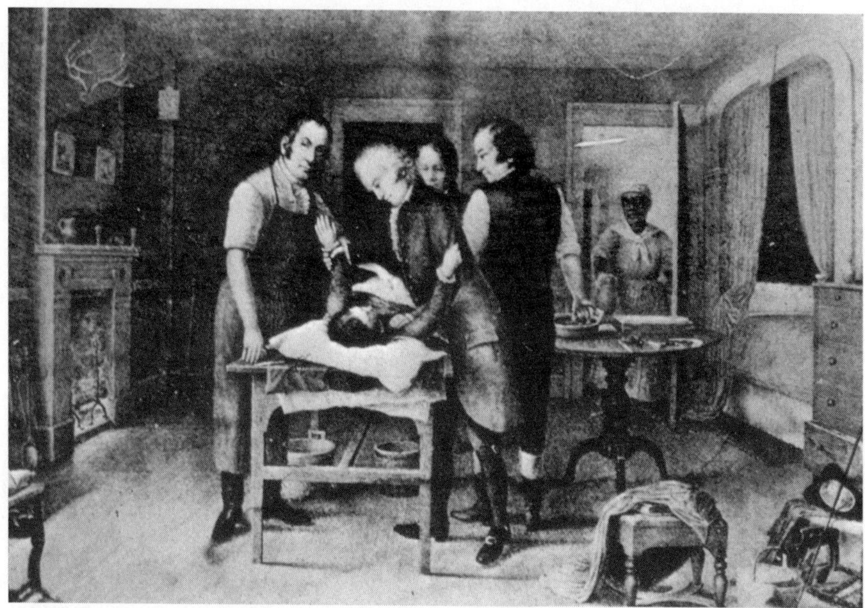

Figure 6: Depiction of McDowell's operation by George Kasson Knapp. Courtesy of McDowell House, Danville, Kentucky.

uterine fibroid from a second patient in 1813, and also excised a six-pound "schirrhous [hardened cancerous] ovarium" from a third patient in 1816, he submitted a report of those three cases to his old mentor at the University of Edinburgh, John Bell. At the time the report reached Scotland, John Bell was away, and therefore it was received by Bell's associate, John Lizars. This submission by McDowell would not be set in print until it was incorporated in a report by Lizars detailing two of his own unsuccessful cases, one in which the tumor was not found and the other in which the patient died without an operative procedure. Lizars's paper appeared in the *Edinburgh Medical Journal* in October 1824, fifteen years after McDowell's seminal operation.[9]

At the same time that McDowell mailed his report to Scotland, a copy was transmitted for him by Dr. William A. McDowell, another of Ephraim's nephews, who spent five years as a pupil and two years as an associate of Ephraim. William McDowell submitted the report to Professor Philip Syng Physick with the author's request that it be published in the *Eclectic Repertory and Analytical Review* "if found worthy." The exact circumstances leading to Physick's assessment of the report and his rejection are unknown.

No written critique was ever offered. It can be speculated that the improbable geographic origin of the report and the lack of recognition of the reporting surgeon played contributory roles.

Following Physick's rejection, William McDowell brought the report to Dr. Thomas Chalkley James, professor of midwifery at the University of Pennsylvania, who was also one of the four editors of the *Eclectic Repertory and Analytical Review.* The paper was accepted by Dr. James and appeared in print in October 1817.[10] A second report, in the form of correspondence to Dr. James from Ephraim McDowell, appeared in the same journal two years later.[11] The contents of that second paper consisted of a description of two additional patients. One patient had a five-pound solid ovarian tumor removed in April 1817, and she recovered. The other patient was operated upon a year later after four episodes in which McDowell had removed over thirteen quarts of gelatinous material from her abdomen by "tapping" (providing drainage). At the operation sixteen quarts of gelatinous material were removed from the tumor and abdomen, but the patient died on the third postoperative day.

McDowell's second report also included a response to criticisms that appeared in the *Eclectic Repertory and Analytical Review* in 1818 directed at the first report. McDowell's two publications constitute the sum total of his contributions to surgical literature. He never published his experience with three additional cases, two of which he deemed to be incomplete removal of ovarian tumors.

The impact of the initial American publication was minimal and of no consequence. One of the published criticisms, which was submitted by Dr. Ezra Michener of Philadelphia, was directed at the lack of details in the first report:

> It is much to be regretted that cases so interesting to the community as those of Dr. McDowell's and as novel as interesting, should come before the public in such a manner as to frustrate the intention of becoming useful.
>
> Far be it from me to arraign the probity of Doctor McDowell. If the cases he relates are, as I sincerely hope them to be, correctly stated, no remarks of mine can detract from their merit.[12]

In another criticism, Dr. Thomas Henderson of the District of Columbia wrote:

> That which was believed to be ovarian disease, was proved not to be so; and if this mode of investigation was more attended to, and even if one writer in

the *Eclectic Repertory*, Doctor McDowell had been more considerate in the examination and detail of his cases, and with all due respect I would suggest that *it is still his duty to be so* something very interesting might have been preserved to the profession on this subject.[13]

McDowell's surgical credo was encapsulated by the response he made to these criticisms:

[A]nd I think my description of the mode of operating, and of the anatomy of the parts concerned, clear enough, to enable any good anatomist, possessing the judgment requisite for a surgeon, to operate with safety. I hope no operator of any other description may ever attempt it. It is my most ardent wish that this operation may remain, to the mechanical surgeon, forever incomprehensible. Such have been the *bane* of the science; intruding themselves into the ranks of the profession, with no other qualification but boldness in undertaking, ignorance of their responsibility, and indifference to the lives of their patients; proceeding according to the special dictates of some author, as mechanical as themselves, they cut and tear with fearless indifference, utterly incapable of exercising any judgment of their own in cases of emergency; and sometimes, without possessing even the slightest knowledge of the anatomy of the parts concerned.

The preposterous and impious attempts of such pretenders, can seldom fail to prove destructive to the patient, and disgraceful to the science. It is by such this noble science has been degraded, in the minds of many, to the rank of an art.[14]

McDowell's operations were eventually brought into international focus by the 1824 publication of John Lizars. The initial reaction to that article was one of sarcasm and negative criticism. Dr. James Johnson, editor of the *London Medical and Chirurgical Review*, in January 1825 wrote:

Passing over the records of surgery, all of which cannot be depended on, we shall come at once to the recent facts, or alleged facts, communicated in this paper by Mr. Lizars. Three cases of ovarian extirpation occurred, it would seem, some years ago in the practice of Doctor McDowell, of Kentucky, which were transmitted to the late John Bell, and fell into the hands of Mr. Lizars. We candidly confess that we are rather skeptical respecting these statements, and we are rather surprised that Mr. Lizars himself should put implicit confidence in them.[15]

Dr. Johnson also referred to McDowell's description of Jane Todd Crawford's making up her bed on the fifth postoperative day and wrote: "We cannot bring ourselves to credit this statement." In the same issue of this journal, Dr. Johnson, in reviewing work by Professor James Blundell, who indicated that there was a future for ovariotomy, wrote:

> In despite all that has been written respecting this cruel operation, we entirely disbelieve that it has ever been performed with success, nor do we think it ever will.[16]

Only twenty months later, in October 1826, the same Dr. Johnson, after reviewing the *North American Medical and Surgical Journal* of that year recanted with the acknowledgment:

> Extirpation of the Ovarium—A back settlement of America—Kentucky—has beaten the mother country, nay, Europe itself, with all the boasted surgeons thereof, in the fearful and formidable operation of gastrotomy (referring to opening the abdomen), with extraction of diseased ovaria.[17]

On the occasion of the unveiling of a memorial monument at the grave site of Ephraim McDowell on May 9, 1879, the Harvard professor of anatomy Oliver Wendell Holmes wrote in Boston:

> I am glad that this great achievement is to be thus publicly claimed for American surgery. Our transatlantic cousins have a microphone which enables them to hear the lightest footsteps of their own discoverers and inventors, but they need a telephone with an ear-trumpet at their end to make them hear anything from our side of the water. . . .
>
> A single thought occurs to me which may help to give this occasion something more than professional significance. Although our political independence of the mother country has been long achieved, our scientific and literary independence has been of much slower growth.
>
> And as we read the inscription on this monument, let us gratefully remember that ever bold, forward stride like this grand triumph of science, skill, and moral courage, tends to bring us out of the present period of tutelage and imitation into that brotherhood and self-reliance which should belong to a people no longer a colony or a province, but a mighty nation.[18]

On the eastern face of the memorial made of Virginia granite shaft, the inscription reads: "Beneath this shaft rests Ephraim McDowell, M.D., the 'Father of Ovariotomy,' who, by originating a great surgical operation, became the benefactor of his race, known and honored throughout the civilized world."

But it would have been equally if not more appropriate to recognize that Ephraim McDowell's operations dramatically demonstrated that the abdominal cavity was no longer to be considered as surgically inviolate. Thus, McDowell is deserving of the more encompassing designation of the Founder of Abdominal Surgery.

CHAPTER 3:

THE BEGINNING OF CLINICAL EXPERIMENTATION: BIRTH OF A SPECIALTY

Medicine includes real experiments which are spontaneous, and are not produced by physicians. Experiment is fundamentally only induced observation.

—Claude Bernard
An Introduction to the Study of Experimental Medicine (1866)

Today, the modern gastroenterologist is mandated to undergo training that extends over five to six years after completion of medical school. The usual three-year residency for internal medicine is supplemented by two to three years focusing on the entire gastrointestinal tract, the liver, the biliary system, and the pancreas. Few would guess that this specialty had an unsophisticated, one might say explosive, beginning on a relatively remote island in the Great Lakes. Gastroenterology was ushered in by a surgeon with no scientific background and an improbable patient with a vacillating interest in serving as the object of prolonged experimentation.

It was during the afternoon of June 6, 1822, that a shot rang out in John Jacob Astor's store, the American Fur Company. The store was located on Mackinac Island in a strait between lakes Huron and Michigan. A trapper's shotgun accidentally went off and the whole charge from the muzzle entered the left upper quadrant of the abdomen of Alexis St. Martin, a nineteen-year-old French Canadian trapper, known as a "voyageur." The military surgeon, William Beaumont, stationed at Fort Mackinac, was called to attend the patient. Thus began an association between a doctor and a patient that extended over twelve years, resulting in the publication of a remarkable book that detailed a series of interrelated clinical experiments on a human and initiated the broader science of gastroenterology.

But before embarking on the genesis of both clinical research and gastroenterology, the biography of the surgeon, William Beaumont, merits attention. It not only emphasizes his lack of preparation for scientific inquiry but also provides insight into the early days of military medicine and community surgical practice.

William Beaumont (fig. 7) was born in Lebanon, Connecticut, in 1785. After being educated in public schools, he moved to the community of Champlain in upstate New York, close to the Canadian border, where he conducted the village school and also tended a store. In 1810, he apprenticed himself to Dr. Benjamin Chandler in St. Albans, Vermont, and two years later he was granted a license by the Third Medical Society of the state of Vermont to practice "physic and surgery." In 1812, the United States declared war on Great Britain, and Beaumont crossed Lake Champlain to Plattsburgh, New York, where part of the United States Army was stationed. In Plattsburgh, he was commissioned as a "surgeon's mate" in the 6th Regiment of the United States infantry.

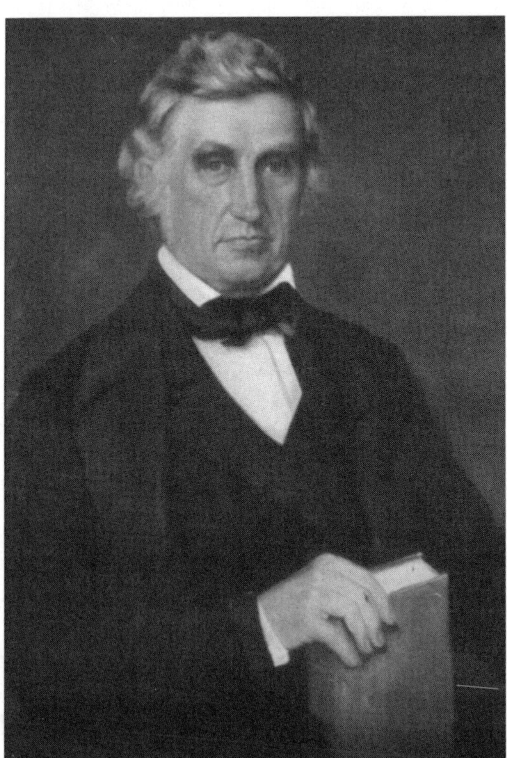

Figure 7: William Beaumont. Courtesy of Becker, Library, Washington University School of Medicine, St. Louis, Missouri.

During the War of 1812, Beaumont tended to the injured troops at the battle at York near Toronto by treating compound fractures, performing three amputations, and a trephination (opening) of the skull. At that battle, the victorious Americans burned the parliament buildings and the governor's mansion. In 1814, the British would retaliate by laying their torches to

Washington, DC, burning the White House and the Capitol building, which, at the time, included the Library of Congress.

Beaumont also participated in the battles at Fort George and Plattsburgh, in New York. Shortly after the Treaty of Ghent was signed, formally ending the War of 1812, Beaumont resigned his commission and entered practice in partnership with another decommissioned army surgeon in Plattsburgh. When Dr. Joseph Lovell was appointed the first surgeon general of the United States Army, he offered Beaumont a position. This led to Beaumont's second commission in the army in December 1819 and his assignment as post physician at Fort Mackinac, on what was then referred to as the northwestern frontier. Beaumont assumed command of the hospital at the fort in June 1820 and carried out all the required military duties.

In keeping with the then current policy, he also received permission to care for the residents of the island's small frontier village, with a population that swelled to as many as five thousand people during the summer when the trappers returned with their furs and pelts. He went on furlough during the summer of 1821 and returned to Plattsburgh to get married. Beaumont then reassumed his island post accompanied by his bride. It was on that remote island in 1822 that he cared for and began his experiments on Alexis St. Martin. The relationship between the investigator and his subject continued at that location until 1825 when Beaumont was transferred to Fort Niagara, in upstate New York. St. Martin's transfer to the post was arranged, but, because he elected to return to his native Canada, no experiments were conducted there.

After slightly more than a year at Fort Niagara, Beaumont was transferred to Fort Howard at Green Bay, a part of the Michigan Territory. In August 1826, he moved on to Fort Crawford at Prairie du Chien on the shore of the upper Mississippi River, where, after an absence of four years, he was joined by Alexis St. Martin, who was specifically brought there by Beaumont so that the experiments could continue.

In 1832, Beaumont participated with the troops in crushing a regional Indian revolt in what is referred to as the Black Hawk War, named after the chief of the Sauk and Fox nations. At the end of the conflict, Beaumont was granted a furlough. After accompanying wounded troops to St. Louis, Missouri, the Beaumont family returned to Plattsburgh, where they were once again joined by Alexis St. Martin. In order to lighten Beaumont's financial burdens, Alexis St. Martin was made sergeant of a detachment of orderlies for which he received compensation. William Beaumont's research on Alexis St. Martin continued, investigating the use of the gastric fistula in the process of digestion. In recognition of that research, the Columbian College of Washington, DC, awarded Beaumont an honorary degree of doctor of medicine in March 1833, prior to publication of his book describing his observations. He was also made an honorary member of the Connecticut Medical Society.

In 1835, Beaumont was transferred from his post in Plattsburgh to Jefferson Barracks, about twelve miles south of St. Louis. Within a year, he had established a lucrative private practice, which, at the time, was permissible for military physicians. St. Louis University established a medical school, and William Beaumont was offered the position as the first chair of surgery. He indicated that he would accept the position if he received permission from the surgeon general, but Beaumont's investiture as the chair never came to pass. In 1839, pending his proposed transfer to a military post in Florida, Beaumont resigned his commission because he had no desire to make the move.

He maintained an active private practice in the area. In 1840, he became the president of the First Medical Society of Missouri, currently the St. Louis Medical Society. In March 1843, he slipped on ice, and although the injury was minor, Beaumont's health deteriorated and he died a month later. In keeping with a commonality that pertains to many stories of America's contributions to surgery, the patient, Alexis St. Martin, outlived the surgeon, in this case by twenty-eight years. St. Martin, the patient-subject, with his persistent gastric fistula (communication between the inside of the stomach and the outside of the overlying skin), did not die until the age of eighty-one, in 1880 (fig. 8).

William Beaumont's monumental scientific contribution is a prime example of the consequence of adhering to the motto "Carpe diem!" The "diem" that was seized brings us back to June 6, 1822, in the American Fur Company store that is still preserved as a historic landmark on Mackinac Island. On that day, the gun that accidentally went off delivered its whole charge, consisting of powder and duck shot, into the left upper abdomen of the young trapper, who was about nineteen years of age. Born Alexis Bidigan, he had since taken the surname St. Martin. The victim lay on the floor with his abdomen penetrated by shot, wadding, and pieces of clothing. William Beaumont was immediately sent for and arrived fifteen minutes later, at which time he found the victim "senseless and apparently in a moribund state."

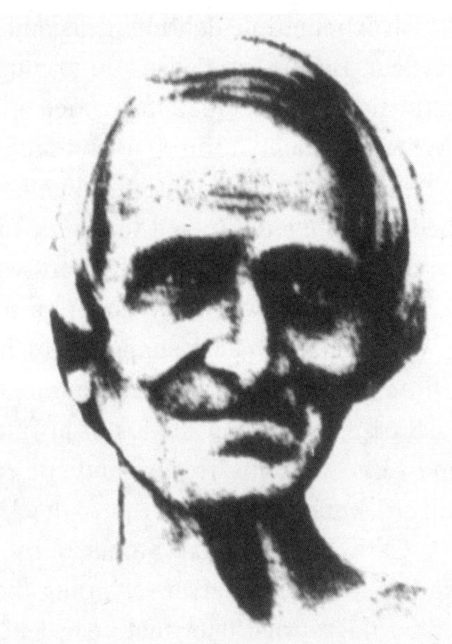

Figure 8: Alexis St. Martin. Courtesy of Becker Library, Washington University School of Medicine, St. Louis, Missouri.

According to Beaumont's own meticulous record, "an area of skin larger than the palm of the hand was blown away, the 5th and 6th ribs were fractured, rupturing the lower portion of the left lobe of the Lungs, and lacerating the Stomach by a spicula of the rib that was blown through it[s] coat. . . . Found a portion of the Lungs as large as a turkey's egg protruding through the external wound, lacerated and burnt, and below this another protrusion resembling the Stomach, . . . with a puncture in the protruding portion large enough to receive my forefinger, and through which a portion of the food that he had taken for breakfast had come out and lodged among his apparel. I considered any attempt to save his life entirely useless."[1]

After the wound was dressed, Alexis St. Martin was moved to a room in the store. Beaumont returned in an hour, removed the destroyed tissue, and cleansed the involved area, "taking away the fragments of the ribs, old flannel wad and the principal charge of shot, all driven together under the skin and into the muscles, and replacing the lungs and stomach as much as possible." He then applied "a carbonated fermenting poultice."[2] St. Martin was then moved to the one-story frame hospital at the fort. For five days a septic fever raged, but on the fifth day the protruding portion of the lung and a piece of the stomach wall sloughed and the patient's fever abated.

For two weeks, before the stomach could retain any material, fluids and nutritional elements were instilled through the anus. St. Martin's appetite then returned, and he was able to take liquids and solid food orally. Beaumont made many attempts to close the opening in the stomach by applying silver nitrate to encourage approximation of the edges of the wounds, but the hole remained open. The patient was a ward of the hospital for about nine months, during which multiple debridements and drainages of wound abscesses were carried out. Beaumont devised a lint plug that was inserted into the stomach and drawn back to occlude the orifice and prevent the loss of oral intake.

When the county refused to continue supporting St. Martin's hospitalization, Beaumont took him into his own home where he "nursed him, fed him, clothed him, lodged him and furnished him with every comfort, and dressed his wounds daily and for the most part twice a day."[3] This was at a time when Beaumont's salary was forty dollars a month and two to four rations daily with which he also had to support his wife and baby daughter.

In the latter half of 1824, Beaumont sent a report of the details of the unusual case and the particulars of his management of it to Surgeon General Joseph Lovell for his review and for permission to publish the material. Lovell submitted the manuscript to the *Medical Recorder*, where it appeared as "A Case of Wounded Stomach by Joseph Lovell, Surgeon General, U.S.A." in 1825.[4] The error regarding the attribution of authorship was corrected by the journal later that year, and, in recognition of the accomplishment, Beaumont was made an honorary member of the Medical Society of Michigan Territory.

Early in 1825, after caring for St. Martin for about two and a half years, Beaumont conceived of the potential for conducting a unique clinical experiment. He noted:

> When he lies on his side I can look directly into the cavity of the Stomach, and almost see the process of digestion. I can pour in water with a funnel, or put in food with a spoon, and draw them out again with a syphon. I have frequently suspended flesh, raw and wasted and other substances into the perforation to ascertain the length of time required to digest each; and at one time used a tent of raw beef, instead of lint to stop the orifice, and found that in less than five hours it was completely digested off, as smooth and even as if it had been cut with a knife.[5]

In an era before ethics committees and institutional review boards, the researcher's concern for the patient is manifest.

> This case affords an excellent opportunity for experimenting upon the gastric fluids and process of digestion. It would give no pain, nor cause the least uneasiness. To extract a gill (pint) of fluid every two or three days, for it frequently flows out spontaneously in considerable quantities. Various

> kinds of digestible substances might be introduced into the stomach, and then easily examined during the process of digestion. I may, therefore, be able hereafter to give some interesting experiments on these subjects.[6]

The first series of four experiments that took place at Fort Mackinac were reported in the *Medical Recorder* in January 1826.[7] The length of time required for digestion of a variety of foods suspended in the stomach by a string was measured. The time of digestion in the stomach was compared with that occurring in vials containing gastric juice. The findings led to the conclusion that gastric juice possessed intrinsic solvents that acted on ingested food. Also, a thermometer that was inserted into the stomach provided measurement of the intragastric temperature.

Because St. Martin seized the opportunity to steal away to Canada during Beaumont's transfer to Fort Niagara in 1825, four years elapsed before the experiments were continued. In 1829, Beaumont was able to track down St. Martin in Canada and arrange to transport him to Fort Crawford in Prairie du Chien, currently in Wisconsin, where Beaumont was posted at the time. It was at that isolated frontier locale where the majority of the experiments were conducted.

Between December 6, 1829, and April 9, 1831, results were recorded for fifty-six experiments, using only a simple thermometer, vials, and a sand bath as laboratory equipment. These included measurements that were made within the stomach during a variety of atmospheric conditions and also during periods of fasting and digestion. Many of the investigations were concerned with the digestibility of various foods. These experiments demonstrated that gastric juice acted as a solvent and that digestion was, in large part, a chemical rather than a physical process.

At this point, Beaumont, with full appreciation of his scientific limitations, felt the need to enlist the assistance of those with an expertise in chemistry. His life as an investigator, however, was interrupted by his participation in the Black Hawk War, at the conclusion of which he was awarded a six-month furlough. He traveled with his family to Plattsburgh, where he met up with St. Martin, who, with Beaumont's permission, had gone to Canada for a brief visit.

On October 16, 1832, an extraordinary covenant was executed. The contract attested to Alexis St. Martin's agreement granting William Beaumont the use of his stomach for experimental purposes.

> It being intended and understood both by said William and said Alexis that the facilities and means afforded by the wounds of the said Alexis in his side and stomach shall be reasonably and properly used and exhibited at all times upon the request or direction of said William for the purposes of science and scientific improvements, the furtherance of knowledge in regard to the power, properties and capacity of the human Stomach.[8]

This probably represents the earliest example of one of the current requisites of an institutional review board prior to the performance of clinical research, the informed consent of the subject.

That year Beaumont traveled to Washington, DC, where he scrupulously reviewed the literature on the physiology of digestion. When he and St. Martin returned to Fort Crawford, an additional series of 116 experiments was conducted between December 1, 1832, and March 1, 1833. During this period, Beaumont established a dialogue with Robley Dunglison, professor of physiology at the University of Virginia, and also with Benjamin Silliman, professor of chemistry at Yale University.

Professor Dunglison, who was Thomas Jefferson's favorite physician, offered Beaumont suggestions for conducting specific experiments and authenticated Beaumont's conclusion that gastric juice contained a significant amount of "muriatic" (hydrochloric) acid and, in addition, acetic acid, along with other constituents that "may never be accurately determined."[9] Professor Silliman added little to the findings and conclusions that Beaumont had made on his own and those incorporating the suggestions of Professor Dunglison.

In July 1833, Beaumont was transferred to Plattsburgh, in accordance with his request, so that the completion of a book incorporating all of his experiments and conclusions could be expedited. St. Martin was awaiting his return, and, between July 9 and November 1, sixty-two additional experiments were performed to confirm previous findings and to determine specifically the time needed to digest different food categories.

The monumental 280-page book, which would be the only medical work included by the Grolier Club as one of the one hundred most important books published in the United States in the nineteenth century, is titled *Experiments and Observations on the Gastric Juice and the Physiology of Digestion.* The first copies, with a dedication to Surgeon General Lovell, came off the press of F. P. Allen, in Plattsburgh, New York, but, because it was initially planned to sell the book by subscription, a "proposal" presenting a synopsis of the work was printed and disseminated in September of that year. Eventually three thousand copies were printed and sold for $3 each. In 2008, a first edition was offered for sale at $3,800, and a copy inscribed by Beaumont was advertised for $35,000.

The narrative of the book, which is accompanied by three engravings depicting the position of the opening into the stomach related to the breast (fig. 9), the aperture into the stomach with the valve depressed, and a portion of the stomach prolapsed through the opening, begins with a chronicle of the accident, the medical care, and the problems of maintaining Alexis St. Martin as the subject of the experiments. Before specifically detailing the experiments, the author offers an expression of humility. That same humility is evidenced in a prior letter that Beaumont wrote to Surgeon General Lovell in his quest of approval:

> A mere tyro in science, with a mind free from every bias, I commenced them, as it were, by accident, and continued desultorily to prosecute them, without regard to any particular arrangement, or the confirmation of anything save plain and palpable truths and physiological facts, aiming singly at the more perfect development of the nature of the Gastric juice and process of Digestion in the human Stomach, subjects which neither time, nor talents, nor labor, nor learning had yet satisfactorily illustrated.
>
> If, in any degree, I succeed in thus contributing to the cause of science, I shall be satisfied with having bestowed my time and patience upon the subject, simply even to afford materials for the Physiologists to cultivate and improve.[10]

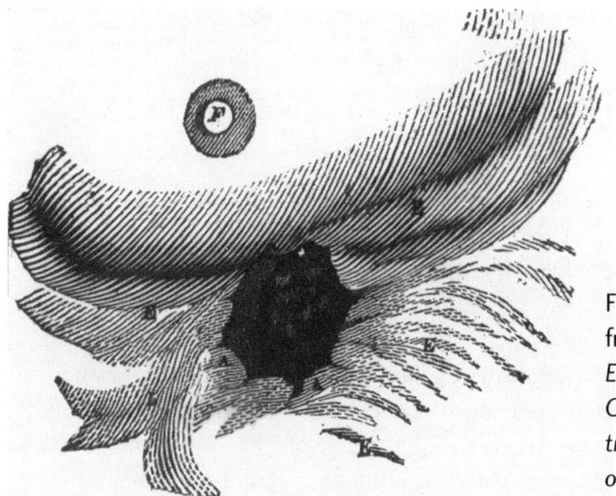

Figure 9: Gastric fistula from William Beaumont's *Experiments and Observations on the Gastric Juice and the Physiology of Digestion* (1833).

After a presentation of the results of his experiments, including a description of the lining of the human stomach, peristalsis within the organ, and the characteristics of gastric juice, Beaumont devotes about one hundred pages to his deductions. This tenacious researcher, without the use of sophisticated laboratory equipment or chemical analyses, was able to conclude several things: digestion occurs within the stomach, where the action of the organ and its juices are basically the same for all foods, but there is a variability with the type and physical characteristics of the food substance; spicy condiments and alcohol ingestion are injurious to the stomach wall; and saliva does not play a significant role in the process of digestion, which begins within the stomach.

Beaumont also demonstrated that the temperature within the stomach is 100 degrees, which may be increased by exercise, decreased by rest, but not altered by digestion per se. He proved that gastric juice is responsible for the digestion of food in the stomach, and that the active agent in gastric juice is muriatic (hydrochloric) acid, which is not found free in the empty stomach. He showed that the secretion of gastric juice is stimulated by the introduction of food or irritants. Pure gastric juice was shown to be clear, acidic, and distinct from mucus. Beaumont also noted that bile secreted by the liver is ordinarily not found in the stomach, is not usually necessary for digestion within the stomach, but does assist when oily foods are ingested. He described the inner surface of the stomach as pale pink and covered by a mucous layer. He indicated that motions of the stomach churn the contents and result in a mixture of food and gastric juice. These motions were both longitudinal (peristalsis) and transverse. Beaumont concluded that the liquid material that leaves the stomach is acted on by bile and pancreatic juice in the duodenum.

The book was well received. The *New York Evening Post* of September 5, 1833, editorialized:

> It will be concluded readily by most men that one of the most important subjects for the study of man is his stomach. In sickness or in health, it equally claims our attention, and the epicure and the dyspeptic are alike engaged, though by many dissimilar modes, in answering the calls or soothing the complaints of this very essential part of the body. We all remember the ingenious apologue on this subject wherein it is shown how the rebellious members were punished for daring to despise and presuming to refuse allegiance to this craving and insatiable monarch. But with all the study that has been bestowed upon this all-important organ and the myste-

> rious powers of digestion, we have been very much in the dark in respect to the causes of its healthful operations or of its morbid actions. Doctors have differed and patients have suffered, while their physicians disputed the reality of gastric juice, or the mysterious region from which all power flows. It seems as if nothing short of a miracle could have enabled man to view the internal operations and test the power of the juices provided by nature to carry on the animal economy; and yet it has been done, and the previous knowledge has been revealed without the aid of miracle, although by a process a little short of one.[11]

In 1838, Sir Andrew Combe, an eminent British physiologist and author of *The Physiology of Digestion Considered in Relation to the Principles of Dietetics* (1841), brought out an English edition of Beaumont's work. In his preface, Combe stresses the importance of the work and expresses his admiration for Beaumont's accomplishments, candor, and humility. But he does state, not in any pejorative way, that Beaumont made no new discovery related to digestion. On the other hand, Combe points out that Beaumont:

> By separating the truth clearly and unequivocally from the numerous errors of fact and opinion with which it was mixed up, and thus converting into certainties points of doctrine in regard to which positive proofs were previously inaccessible, he has given to what was doubtful or imperfectly known a fixed and positive value which it never had before, and which, being once obtained, goes far to furnish us with a clear, connected and consistent view of the general process and laws of digestion.[12]

Unfortunately, current medical students and physicians are usually not acquainted with the name or contributions of William Beaumont, who is simply memorialized on the remote island where the saga began. Near the old officer's quarters at Fort Mackinac, a monument is inscribed with the words: "Near this spot Dr. William Beaumont, U. S. A., made those experiments upon St. Martin which brought fame to himself and honor to American medicine. Erected by the Upper Peninsular and Michigan State medical societies, June 10, 1900." To that we should add Beaumont's credo that found expression in his persistent, careful, and deliberate work. "Truth, like beauty, when unadorned, is adorned the most, and, in prosecuting these experiments and enquiries, I believe I have been guided by its light."[13]

CHAPTER 4:

FOCUS ON FEMALES

A determining point in the history of gynecology is to be found in the fact that sex plays a more important part in the life of woman than in that of man, and that she is more burdened by her sex.

—Henry Sigerist

American Journal of Obstetrics and Gynecology (1941)

Coursing chronologically through the history of the advances in surgery that took place on American soil, the next major breakthrough occurred far from the more sophisticated and acknowledged urban academic establishments. At a time when Philadelphia, Boston, and New York vied for surgical supremacy, the next significant contribution took place at another improbable location. The locale remained relatively rural, in Montgomery, Alabama, well removed from Ephraim McDowell's home west of the Allegheny Mountains and William Beaumont's military posts on Mackinac Island and Prairie du Chien. At the time of this surgical breakthrough, the city of Montgomery, named for the colonial General Richard Montgomery, who was killed during an unsuccessful assault on Quebec in 1775 and is memorialized in a painting by John Trumbull, had a population of less than thirty thousand.

The accomplishment that brought accolades from both sides of the Atlantic Ocean was, simply stated, a purely technical feat. The responsible surgeon, J. Marion Sims (fig. 10), was born in 1813 about a mile from Hanging Rock Creek on the road between Camden and Lancaster, South Carolina—the location that prides itself as the birthplace of President Andrew Jackson and the state that laid claim to the Revolutionary War hero the "Swamp Fox," General Francis Marion, from whom Sims's middle name derived. After the family moved to Lancaster and Sims completed his early education at the Franklin Academy, he entered the junior class at South Carolina College, which later became the University of South Carolina in

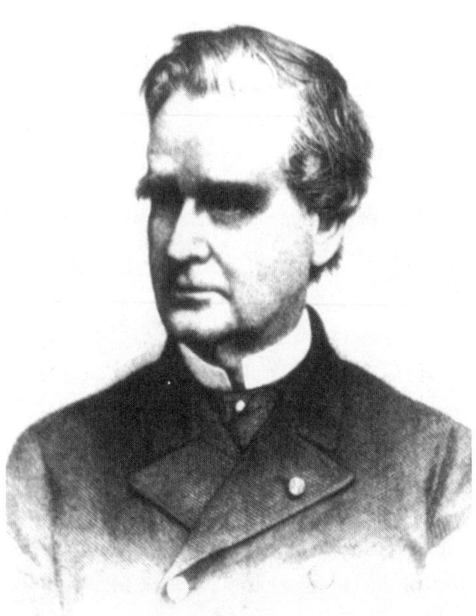

Figure 10: J. Marion Sims. Courtesy of Edward G. Miner Library University of Rochester School of Medicine and Dentistry, Rochester, New York.

Columbia. He graduated in 1832 with a BA and, much to his father's disappointment, decided on a career in medicine. Following the usual course, Sims initially associated himself with a local physician, Dr. Churchill Jones, and then, in order to gain some rudimentary introduction, completed a fourteen-week course in medicine at the newly established Medical College of South Carolina, generally referred to as the Charleston Medical School.

Sims selected a relatively new school in Philadelphia, Jefferson Medical College, which was established in 1825, to complete his medical education. His selection was predicated on the fact that, unlike the more-renowned University of Pennsylvania, the school had a history of attracting students from the South, and it was recognized for the surgical prowess of one of its founders, Dr. George McClellan. Early evidence of Sims's manual dexterity is attested to by his being singled out to assist Dr. McClellan at operations. An interesting vignette Sims recalled in his autobiography recounts his giving to the four- or five-year-old son of the professor of surgery "sixpences to buy ginger bread and taffy."[1] That little boy went on to become General George B. McClellan, one of the commanding generals of the Union Army during the Civil War and the Democratic Party's unsuccessful candidate for the presidency in 1864. Sims received his doctor of medicine degree in 1835.

With diploma in hand, Sims returned to Lancaster, where he rented an office and hung a shingle that read "J. Marion Sims, Physician and Surgeon." Unfortunately, the first two patients he treated were moribund septic babies who died under his care. This prompted his move to Alabama, which, at the time, was attracting many Carolinians. He practiced for a brief period in

Mount Meigs and Cubahatchee, and then settled in Montgomery toward the end of 1840, six years before that city became the state capital.

It was in Montgomery that a drama would unfold and launch the career of Sims in the realm of gynecologic surgery. During the first four years of his practice in Montgomery, Sims developed his reputation as a surgeon. He was the first in the South to successfully treat clubfoot and also strabismus (lack of parallelism of the visual axis of the eyes). His successful management of a patient with "hare lip" (cleft lip and palate) resulted in his first publication, an article that appeared in the *American Journal of Dental Science.*[2]

But the saga that was central to Sims's professional persona began in June 1845 when he participated in a forceps delivery of the baby of a seventeen-year-old plantation slave, whose name was Anarcha. As a consequence of the prolonged labor and the extraction of the baby, Anarcha developed a vesicovaginal fistula and a rectovaginal fistula (abnormal passages between the bladder and the rectum with the vagina, respectively), making her unfit for her plantation duties. This was the first time that Sims had encountered a patient with a vesicovaginal fistula. It had transformed the young lady into a social pariah because of the constant perineal (the region between the genital organs and the anus) soiling. Although rare surgical successes had been reported as anecdotes, at the time, the disorder was generally considered to be untreatable.

Coincidentally, shortly thereafter, Sims was asked to see another seventeen-year-old slave, Betsey, and, subsequently, eighteen-year-old Lucy, both with vesicovaginal fistulas that precluded their acting as house servants. In order to expedite examination of the fistulous opening, Sims inserted a bent spoon handle into the vagina to allow the ingress of air and dilation of the canal. The improved visualization of the fistula was so encouraging that Sims "ransacked the country for cases" and added a second story to his small hospital so that twelve patients could be housed. He contracted with the owners of the slaves, indicating that he would keep and feed the patients if the owners would pay their taxes and clothe them. Unfortunately, the young women were regarded as property and therefore could not sign permission granting informed consent.

The situation was, however, to some degree analogous to the circumstance that pertained to William Beaumont, being presented a medical problem that demanded attention and allowed experimentation. Sims also seized the day and sought the opportunity to care for several patients with a dreadful disorder on whom he could experiment in attempt to effect a cure. It is particularly interesting that Sims writes in his autobiography that before he saw his first case of vesicovaginal fistula, "I never pretended to treat any diseases of women, and if any woman came to consult me on account of any functional derangement of the uterine system, I immediately replied, 'This is out of my line, I don't know anything about it practically.'"[3]

The surgical plan was to excise the edges of the fistula within the vagina, bring the new edges of the vaginal surface together with sutures, and drain the bladder with a catheter until the healing was complete. It took three weeks to have the necessary instruments made, including a proper speculum that was constructed of German steel, with a seven-inch handle and a two-and-a-half-inch concave end to be positioned in the vagina. The concavity was polished so that it would optimally reflect the sunlight, which was focused in the vagina by means of a small mirror.

In December 1845, Lucy was the first patient operated upon. During the procedure, her pain and that experienced by all of the patients was blunted only by opiates, because Sims, like essentially the entire surgical world, had no knowledge of surgical anesthesia.

Sims did not know that three years previously, less than three hundred miles away in Georgia, Dr. Crawford W. Long had used the inhalation of sulfuric ether to obviate pain while he operated on patients. But Dr. Long did not publish his experience with several patients until the report of similar success at the Massachusetts General Hospital appeared in 1846. Decades later, when Sims enjoyed a vaunted position in surgery, his article on the "Discovery of Anesthesia" in the May 1877 issue of the *Virginia Medical Monthly* set off his campaign to credit Dr. Long with the discovery of surgical anesthesia.[4]

The first operation, performed to close Lucy's fistula, failed. Similarly, operations on Betsey and Anarcha, in that order, were also unsuccessful. In spite of multiple technical modifications, years of continuous frustration ensued for Sims. Failure followed failure to achieve permanent, complete closure of the fistula in any of the patients, despite several operations on each. Fortunately, no patient died, and only one sustained a serious infection.

Eventually, Sims speculated that the failures might be attributable to the silk sutures being employed to bring the edges of the fistula together. After failing with lead sutures, he had the local jeweler make wire of pure silver about the width of a horsehair. In May 1849, almost four years after he had participated in her forceps delivery, Sims operated once again on Anarcha.

This represented her thirtieth procedure without anesthesia. As Sims would later write in his autobiography:

> The operation was performed on the fistula in the base of the bladder, that would admit the end of my little finger; she had been cured on one fistula in the base of the bladder. The edges of the wound were nicely denuded, and neatly brought together with four of these fine silver wires. They were passed through little strips of lead, one on one side of the fistula, and the other on the other. The sutures was tightened, and then secured or fastened by the perforated shot run on the wire, and pressed with forceps to avoid loosening.[5]

Anarcha's fistula remained closed, encouraging Sims to repeat the procedure on Lucy, Betsey, and the others in his care. Working at a feverish pace, success followed success in every instance, and no untoward incident occurred. Sims's experience was reported in an article titled "Treatment of Vesicovaginal Fistula" in the *American Journal of Medical Sciences* in 1852.[6] Thus, the medical world was informed of a major breakthrough in the treatment of a devastatingly compromising condition.

It is now appreciated that wire sutures, currently made of stainless steel, evoke less reaction from surrounding tissues than silk, and that braided silk consists of minute interstices that provide sites for the development of local infection by bacteria in those areas.

Because of recurrent attacks of severe and disabling diarrhea that he thought might be related to the hot weather, Sims elected to leave the South and settle permanently in New York City. In the summer of 1853, the Sims family occupied a home at 79 (appears as 89 in Sims's autobiography) Madison Avenue between Twenty-eighth and Twenty-ninth streets. Initially, he was unable to attract patients. But shortly after his arrival, Sims was referred a case by Dr. Valentine Mott, who was the most notable surgeon in the city and for whom the chair of surgery at Columbia University Presbyterian Hospital currently is named. Sims successfully repaired a vesicovaginal fistula in the patient as Dr. Mott and his son, also a surgeon, observed. This was the first time a vesicovaginal fistula was cured in New York.

Several New York City surgeons adopted the technique and achieved similar success. The competitive atmosphere precluded Sims from operating at the major hospitals and stimulated him to create his own hospital for the treatment of disorders of women. With the support of some women among the social elite and endorsements from three influential medical leaders—

including Dr. Valentine Mott, the president of the College of Physicians and Surgeons, and also the president of the New York Medical College—a charter for a hospital was secured.

The Woman's Hospital opened its doors at 83 Madison Avenue between Twenty-third and Twenty-fourth streets on May 1, 1855. It constituted the first hospital in the United States dedicated solely to the care of medical ailments exclusive to women. If one discounts the Rotunda Obstetric Hospital in Dublin, Ireland, it was the first such hospital in the world. Initially, the hospital contained about thirty beds, and most of the patients were charity cases. At the onset, a few beds were reserved for prosperous patients and those of modest means.

The patient population was a stimulus for Sims to develop new instruments, such as uterine elevators, and a method to easily remove uterine polyps, one that soon became standard in other hospitals. Each year as many as five hundred medical professionals would observe Sims perform his operations. The Woman's Hospital attracted so many women from all over the country with a wide variety of disorders unique to the female gender that the need for expansion soon became apparent. Consequently, in anticipation of building a new and more expansive hospital, a charter was obtained in 1857 for the Woman's Hospital of the State of New York.

The land selected for the new hospital was located between Forty-ninth and Fiftieth streets, and Lexington and Fourth (currently Park) avenues. This is now the site of the Waldorf-Astoria Hotel. Before that hospital could be built, however, twenty-seven thousand corpses had to be exhumed from what had served as the old Potter's Field during the cholera epidemic of 1832 and reburied on Ward's Island in New York City's East River. The building of the hospital was further delayed by the Civil War, but the doors did finally open in 1867. That hospital was later replaced by a larger building at 119th Street on New York City's Upper West Side.

The fall of Fort Sumter in Sims's home state and the onset of the Civil War created in him a sense of discomfort as a Southerner working in the North. His solution was to go abroad, and he set out unaccompanied by his family in 1861. In Dublin, his first port of call, he was warmly welcomed and while there he successfully demonstrated the technique that he had developed for repair of a vesicovaginal fistula. After visiting Edinburgh and London, Sims proceeded to Paris, where he was particularly regaled for successfully closing several vesicovaginal fistulas before distinguished surgical audiences.

After an absence of six months, he returned to New York, and, in July 1862, the entire Sims family moved to Paris so he could apply his medical talents while waiting out the American conflict. Sims's reputation took him all over Europe and allowed him to provide medical services to the Duchess of Hamilton and Empress Eugénie of France. The Sims family later moved to London, and, in the latter half of 1864, Great Britain's most influential journal, the *Lancet*, published a series of articles by J. Marion Sims under the title of "Clinical Notes on Uterine Surgery, with Special Reference to the Management of Sterile Conditions."[7] These publications appeared in book form two years later and serve as testimony to the fact that Sims might be regarded as the first American reproductive biologist or sterility specialist. He accurately described a postcoital test for the presence and viability of sperm. Sims demonstrated that spermatozoa entered cervical mucus rapidly, and that they could remain there for forty-eight hours.[8]

After a prolonged stay in Europe that extended over seven years and was characterized by the acquisition of large surgical fees and honors from royalty, Sims and his family returned to New York City. For the remainder of his life, Sims shuttled back and forth between the United States and Europe. In New York, he continued as a member of the Woman's Hospital medical board until December 1, 1874, when Sims was provoked to tender his resignation, which was accepted.

Two issues sparked this unanticipated action. The nonmedical board of governors limited the number of spectators at any one operation to fifteen, whereas Sims's operations frequently attracted double that number of spectators. For Sims, the other intolerable condition was the board's ruling that no patient with uterine cancer could be admitted to the hospital, probably because of the repugnant odor associated with the tumors.

A decade later, two month's before he died, Sims wrote a letter urging the establishment of a hospital for the exclusive treatment of cancer in women. Three months after his death, the cornerstone was laid for the Astor Pavilion of the New York Cancer Hospital. Ten years later a pavilion was added for men. The center is now known as the Memorial Sloan-Kettering Cancer Center.

Sims morphed into the role of an esteemed elder statesman as evidenced by his election to the presidency of the American Medical Association in 1875, only a few months after his resignation from the Woman's Hospital. Those who were responsible for his election indicated that it represented a strong endorsement of his stand as a physician against a nonprofessional governing board of a hospital. In 1881, as a rapprochement, Sims was appointed to the post of senior consulting surgeon at the Woman's Hospital.

Outside the realm of gynecology, in 1878, while in Paris, Sims performed the first planned operation on the gallbladder. The patient died eight days later. (This pioneering effort is more appropriately considered in chapter 6. Our current emphasis is on Sims's gynecologic accomplishments that earned him the appellation Father of Modern Gynecology.) Sims was elected president of the American Gynecological Society in 1880, three years before he died.

J. Marion Sims was buried in a Brooklyn cemetery. He is memorialized by a monument on the grounds of the South Carolina state capitol, and in Columbia, the city where he received his baccalaureate degree. In Lancaster, a hospital bears his name. A full-length statue honors him on the capitol grounds in Montgomery, Alabama, where Sims's revolutionary operations were performed. In Sims's adopted city of New York, in Central Park at Fifth Avenue and 103rd Street, appropriately opposite the New York Academy of Medicine, stands the most impressive of his memorial statues, accompanied by a description of his accomplishments, chiseled in marble.

But these statues now attract little attention from passersby. Thousands of disinterested pedestrians, particularly in New York City, rarely look at the figure, and fewer still read the inscriptions. Currently, few in the public at large appreciate who the man was or the magnitude of his accomplishments. Rather, historians and sociologists have shined a light on Sims's major accomplishment with a contentious coda that has been included in recognition afforded him in the *American National Biography*.[9]

In the late twentieth century's appraisals of the male attitude toward women and racial issues, Sims is attacked for operating without anesthesia on black female slaves who had no claim to decision making about their bodies. G. J. Barker-Benfield, the author of *The Horrors of the Half-Known Life*, fervently castigates Sims:

> It was women who were first selected as a group for surgical innovation, their bodies the field and the contending parties the surgeons. The [Woman's] hospital patients were treated free; Sims and the other gynecological surgeons made their money by applying the hospital discoveries in private practice, where they charged stupendous fees. The conclusion is inescapable that the hospital was instituted for the same reason that Sims

> garnered diseased black women into his backyard—to provide guinea pigs for his self-education, before he and the others could convincingly offer care to the wives of the wealthy who were originally Sims's backers for the hospital.[10]

In an article that was published in *Sage: A Scholarly Journal on Black Women*, in 1985, the author concludes that

> Sims failed utterly to recognize his patients as autonomous persons, and his own personal drive for success cannot be minimized, especially as a balance to the enormous amount of praise accorded Sims for his work.[11]

Nevertheless, it must be remembered that the only patients with vesicovaginal fistulas whom Sims saw initially were black slaves and that these women were afflicted with a disorder that made them social outcasts. Surgical anesthesia had not been widely appreciated at the time. It is purely speculative that the Woman's Hospital, which was actually established to provide care for women who could not afford it, was constructed as an experimental laboratory. The era of Sims's achievements surely did not embody the social conscience of today. Informed consent had not been developed, but there is nothing to suggest that the patients did not agree to serve as experimental subjects when the hope of cure was a possibility.

Whether Sims was a boon to society or a beast may be a subject for argument, but his contributions to the care of women were monumental and cannot be contested.

CHAPTER 5:

THE DEATH OF PAIN

The extraordinary controversy which has raged, and re-raged every few years, on the question to whom the world is indebted for the introduction of anaesthesia, illustrates the absence of true historical perspective, and a failure to realize just what priority means in the case of a great discovery.

—Sir William Osler
Remarks on presenting William Morton's papers to the Royal Society of Medicine (May 15, 1918)

As the first half of the nineteenth century was coming to an end, surgical procedures had emphasized speed in order to minimize the period of extreme pain. Amputations, the most commonly performed major operations, were carried out in mere minutes. Baron Larrey, Napoleon's surgeon—whose name appears on the Arc de Triomphe and who is honored by interment with Napoleon at Les Invalides—could disarticulate the shoulder joint in one minute and had performed two hundred amputations in one day on the battlefield at the battle of Borodino in 1812. The British surgeon Robert Liston would amputate a leg in two minutes. Patients would rely on prayers, singing, and mesmerism for distraction. A fortunate few had the pain blunted by whiskey, dilaudid, or opium.

Then came what is generally regarded to be the United States' most significant contribution to surgery—surgical anesthesia. It has been said that surgical anesthesia is the greatest discovery of humankind. Frank Kells Boland, professor of clinical surgery at Emory University, wrote: "[To] the individual who has experienced the power of surgical anesthesia to prevent pain, restore health, and save life, all other human contributions become secondary in comparison."[1]

Currently, one of the highlights offered by the Boston Chamber of Commerce is the "Innovation Odyssey," a guided tour that includes a visit to the

Ether Dome in the Bulfinch Building of Massachusetts General Hospital. The cornerstone of the building was laid on July 4, 1818. Between 1821 and 1868, about eight thousand operations were performed in what was then known as the surgical amphitheater. Since the event that took place on October 16, 1846, the amphitheater has been referred to as the "Ether Dome," which in 1965 was declared a National Historic Site. It was completely restored, albeit incorporating modern amenities, in time for the anniversary of the first successful demonstration of the efficacy of ether anesthesia for surgical procedures. Electric lights have replaced the original natural illumination through a glass roof, and the original seven rows of wooden benches have given way to six tiers of metal seats. Modern telecommunication and audiovisual equipment have also been incorporated.

On October 16, 1846, in the surgical amphitheater of the Bulfinch Building, the first public demonstration of surgical anesthesia took place. On that day, painless surgery was born. The featured players in the drama were William Thomas Green Morton as the anesthetist, John Collins Warren as the surgeon, and Edward Gilbert Abbott as the patient. Although there is no argument that surgical anesthesia should be credited to American efforts, the story of the inception of this seminal contribution is both convoluted and contentious. It is a saga featuring dramatic events and a curious cast of characters whose lives after the discovery were enveloped by tragedy.

Ether, the anesthetic agent, had been known and considered for potential use for almost six centuries before its surgical application. Ether was discovered in 1275 by the Spanish chemist Raymundus Lullius (Raymond Lully), who called it "sweet oil of vitriol," and was synthesized in 1540 by the German chemist Valerius Cordus. Also in the sixteenth century, the first hint of the potential of ether as an anesthetic agent was expressed by the famous Swiss alchemist, physician, astronomer, and occultist Theophrast Phillipus Aureolus Bombastus von Hohenheim, who conveniently took the name Paracelsus (the equal of Celsus, the author of *De Medicina*, who lived in Rome between 25 BCE and 50 CE). Paracelsus said, "It [ether] quiets all suffering and relieves all pain."[2] The name "Aether" was first applied to the chemical by German scientist Wilhelmus Godofredus Frobenius in 1730. The initial medical applications were as treatment for phthisis (tuberculosis), other pulmonary problems, and bladder stones.

Ether, as an agent to induce inhalation anesthesia, was preceded by nitrous oxide, which was first made in 1772 by Joseph Priestley, better known for his discovery of the gas that was later named oxygen. At the end of the eighteenth century, the brilliant English scientist Humphry Davy experimented with nitrous oxide and stated in his work titled *Researches, Chemical and Philosophical, Chiefly concerning Nitrous Oxide* (1800):

> As nitrous oxide in its extensive operation appears capable of destroying physical pain, it may probably be used with advantage during surgical operations in which no great effusion of blood takes place.[3]

The first member of the medical profession to vigorously champion the cause of inhalation anesthesia was Henry Hill Hickman, who practiced medicine and surgery in Shropshire, England. He published an extraordinary pamphlet in 1824 in which he reported a series of surgical procedures, including amputations of the limbs of mice and dogs and the ears of rabbits, using carbon dioxide to obviate pain. He proposed that the procedure should be applied to humans as well.[4]

Less than two decades later, the locale for the application of surgical anesthesia shifted to the United States, where it rapidly became a reality. Although the definitive drama of discovery took place in Boston, the first use of ether as an anesthetic agent, and the first application of inhalation anesthesia to suppress pain during a surgical procedure, must be credited to Dr. Crawford W. Long (fig. 11), a twenty-six-year-old physician practicing in Jefferson, Georgia, a community of several hundred inhabitants about eighteen miles from the city of Athens, Georgia.

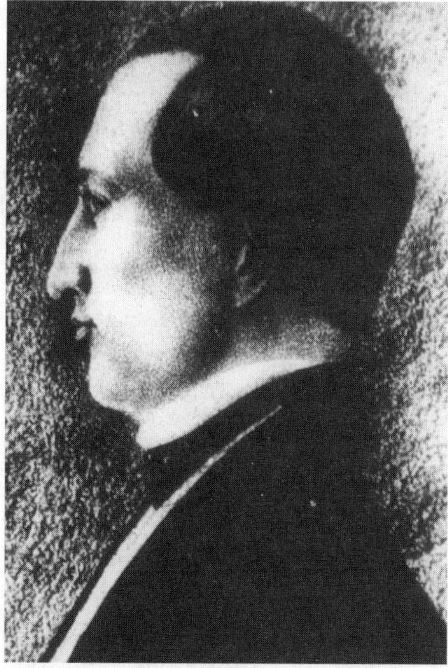

Figure 11: Dr. Crawford W. Long. Courtesy Edward G. Miner Library, University of Rochester School of Medicine and Dentistry, Rochester, New York.

Long was a native Georgian, who, after graduating Franklin College (later to become the University of Georgia), matriculated at the medical department of Transylvania University at Lexington, Kentucky. He later transferred to the University of Pennsylvania, where he received his medical degree in 1839. While in Philadelphia, Long learned of the "laughing parties" based on the soporific effects of both nitrous oxide and ether, which led to application of surgical anesthesia. After visiting the distinguished hospitals in New York City for eighteen months, he opened his office.

On March 30, 1842, Long administered ether during an operation in which two small tumors were removed from the neck of James M. Venable. The ether was given by means of a soaked towel that was placed on the nose and the mouth. The patient remained asleep during the procedure and experienced no pain. Two months later another tumor was removed from the back of the neck of the "etherized" Venable. Long administered ether on another occasion that year when he amputated a toe of a young boy.

Long did not report his experiences until he learned of the event that took place in Boston and read several reports on the use of sulphuric ether "for the purpose of rendering patients insensible during surgical operations." Long eventually reported his experiences in detail in the *Southern Medical and Surgical Journal* of December 1849.[5] That report included the sworn testimony of the patient Mr. Venable and the mother of the child who had his toe amputated, along with written statements by those who witnessed the procedures. If we accept the authority of the latest edition of the *Oxford English Dictionary*, the first definition of "discoverer" is "one who first finds out that which was previously unknown," which makes Long the incontestable discoverer of surgical anesthesia.

Long, however, never participated as a claimant for the discovery of surgical anesthesia. Few were acquainted with the article he published in a relatively obscure journal, but he did have his advocates. In May 1877, an article titled "Discovery of Anesthesia" appeared in the *Virginia Medical Monthly*.[6] That article, written by the highly esteemed medical personality J. Marion Sims, championed Long's contribution. Sims insisted that credit for the discovery must first go to Long, next to Horace Wells, and thereafter to W. T. G. Morton and Charles T. Jackson. Sims suggested that Congress grant a stipend to all four men or their surviving families.

The *Johns Hopkins Hospital Bulletin* of 1897 includes an article by the famous urologist Hugh H. Young titled "Long, the Discoverer of Anesthesia: A Presentation of the Original Documents."[7] The author, in addition to crediting Long with the discovery, also alleges that when King Edward VII awoke from the anesthetic that was administered during the draining of his appendiceal abscess, he asked his surgeon, Sir Frederick Treves, "Who discovered anesthesia?" Treves replied that it was an American, Dr. Crawford W. Long. Long is honored with a medallion that was produced by his alma mater, the University of Pennsylvania, in 1912; a statue in Statuary Hall in the nation's capitol, and a hospital that bears his name in Atlanta, Georgia.

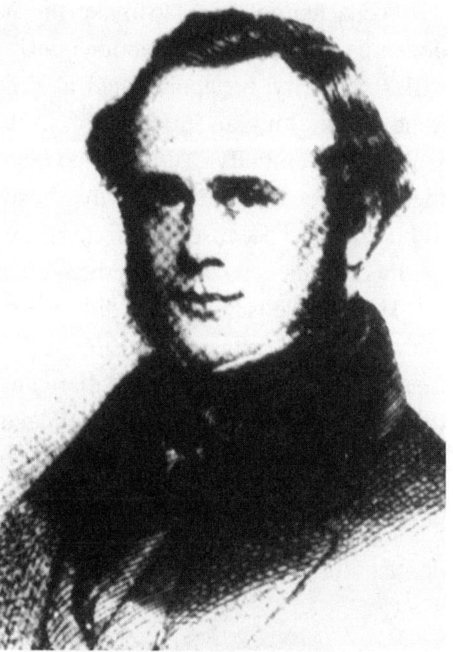

Figure 12: Horace Wells. Courtesy of Massachusetts General Hospital Archives and Special Collections.

Horace Wells (fig. 12) was the first to enter the stage in the dramatic saga that eventually took place at the "Ether Dome" of Massachusetts General Hospital, and he is accorded an element of priority among the tragic troika—those who staked a claim for discovery of surgical anesthesia. Wells's story begins on the evening of December 11, 1844, in Hartford, Connecticut. During a private exhibition that was conducted specifically for entertainment to demonstrate the "hilarious" effects of "nitrous oxide, Exhilarating or Laughing Gas," one of the volunteer subjects fell and sustained several severe bruises while he was under the influence of inhaled nitrous oxide. When the subject recovered from the effects of the gas, he indicated that he had felt no pain while incurring the bruises. On the occasion, Wells, who had witnessed the event, suggested that an individual could undergo a surgical operation under the influence of the gas and experience no pain.

Wells, a dentist, indicated that he believed that a person could have a tooth extracted painlessly under the influence of nitrous oxide, and, if the demonstrator would administer the gas, he would submit to having his bothersome wisdom tooth extracted by his colleague Dr. Riggs. The proposal came to fruition and painless dentistry was born!

Wells learned how to make the gas and proceeded to perform over a dozen painless dental extractions during the ensuing month. In order to gain wider publicity, he approached a former student and dental partner in the hope of soliciting an introduction to the surgeons of Massachusetts General Hospital. Eventually, Wells carried out a demonstration of nitrous oxide anesthesia for dental extraction at that hospital in January 1845, but it turned out to be a failure because no anesthesia was achieved and his method was discredited in the eyes of his medical colleagues.

Horace Wells, however, did receive recognition posthumously. In 1864, the American Dental Association declared Wells to be the discoverer of anesthesia. Four years later, the American Medical Association resolved: "That the honor of the discovery of practical anesthesia is due to the late Dr. Horace Wells, of Connecticut." This was formally affirmed in 1872. In the Place des États Unis, near the Arc de Triomphe, is a bust inscribed: "Au dentiste Americain Horace Wells inovateur de l'anesthesie chirurgical" (To the American dentist Horace Wells, innovator of the surgical anesthesia).

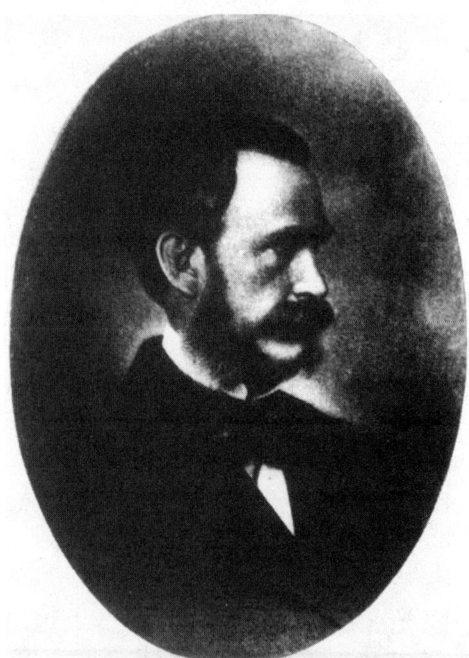

Figure 13: William Thomas Green Morton. Courtesy of Massachusetts General Hospital Archives and Special Collections.

If we accept the precept stated by Sir Francis Darwin in *Eugenics Review* in 1914 that "in science credit goes to the man who convinces the world, not to the man to whom the idea first occurs," then William Thomas Green Morton is to be credited with the establishment of surgical anesthesia. Morton (fig. 13), a student and partner of Horace Wells, attended the first independent college of dentistry in Baltimore and specialized in prosthetic dentistry that frequently required removal of multiple teeth from a single patient—a painful procedure that was a deterrent for many prospective clients. For Morton's practice, anesthesia represented a poten-

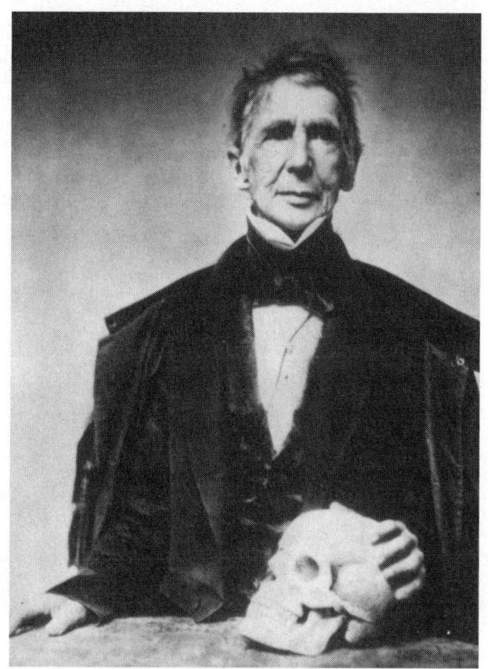

Figure 14: John Collins Warren. Courtesy of Massachusetts General Hospital Archives and Special Collections.

tial boon that would stimulate patients to accept the procedures. In 1844, Morton first used the local application of liquid ether at the suggestion of Charles T. Jackson to reduce the pain associated with filling a tooth. He then began to experiment with the use of inhaled ether as a topical anesthetic agent or with inhalation as a method of administration.

Once Morton gained confidence with his capability to produce insensibility and obviate pain during a surgical procedure, he sought the opportunity to demonstrate and advertise his achievement. What better stage than the Harvard Medical School? Morton approached Dr. John Collins Warren (fig. 14), who was one of the founders of Massachusetts General Hospital in 1811 and who followed his father as the second professor of anatomy and surgery at Harvard Medical School. Morton purposefully did not reveal specifics about the agent to be used because he anticipated applying for a patent. Warren agreed to participate in the demonstration by conducting an operation, which was scheduled for October 16, 1846, at 10 AM. At the appointed hour, those assembled in the surgical amphitheater included the patient, Gilbert Abbott; the operating surgeon, John Collins Warren; the surgeon, Henry J. Bigelow, who is credited with orchestrating the event; and other members of the surgical staff. Morton was delayed, awaiting last-minute changes that were being made by a Mr. Chamberlain, who produced the ether inhaler that was to be used.

The apparatus (fig. 15) consisted of a glass globe with two ports that contained an ether-soaked sea sponge. One port allowed the addition of liquid sulphuric ether that vaporized within the globe. The other port contained the

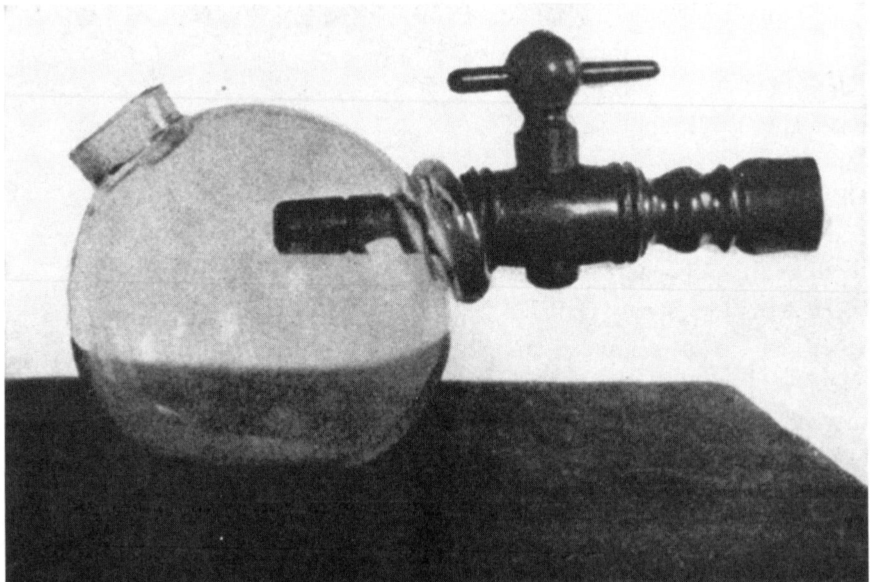

Figure 15: The original inhaler used by Morton. Courtesy of Massachusetts General Hospital Archives and Special Collections.

breathing device. The brass cylinder that connected the globe with the mouthpiece incorporated a leather flap valve that opened on inspiration and closed at the beginning of expiration, thereby creating unidirectional flow. The subject held the mouthpiece in his lips while his nasal passages were held closed.

After waiting for fifteen minutes beyond the appointed hour, Warren was about to proceed without anesthesia when Morton arrived and was greeted by Warren with the statement, "Well sir! Your patient is ready." After administering the ether, Morton countered, "Your patient it ready." The operation then took place. Warren described the event:

> The patient was a young man, about twenty years old, having a tumor on the left side of the neck, lying parallel to and just below the left portion of the lower jaw. . . . The patient was arranged in a sitting posture, and everything made ready. . . . The patient was then made to inhale a fluid from a tube connected with a glass globe. After four or five minutes he appeared to be asleep, and was thought by Dr. Morton to be in a condition for the operation. I made an incision between two and three inches long in the direction of the tumor, and to my great surprise without any starting, crying or other

> indication of pain . . . and in truth I was not satisfied, until I had, soon after the operation and on various other occasions, asked the question whether he had suffered pain. To this he always replied in the negative, adding, however, he knew of the operation, and comparing the stroke of the knife to that of a blunt instrument passed roughly across his neck.[8]

At the end of the operation, Warren turned to the audience and exclaimed his famous declaration: "Gentlemen, this is no humbug!" (fig. 16).

Shortly thereafter, other operations, including the removal of a fatty tumor from an arm and an amputation, were performed on anesthetized patients at the same hospital. The first paper detailing the experiences was reported by Bigelow on November 9, 1846, at a meeting of the Boston Society of Medical Improvement. Copies of the paper were printed almost simultaneously in the journal of the American Society of Arts and Sciences, the *Boston Medical and Surgical Journal*, and in the *Boston Daily Advertiser* on November 18 and December 9 of that year.[9]

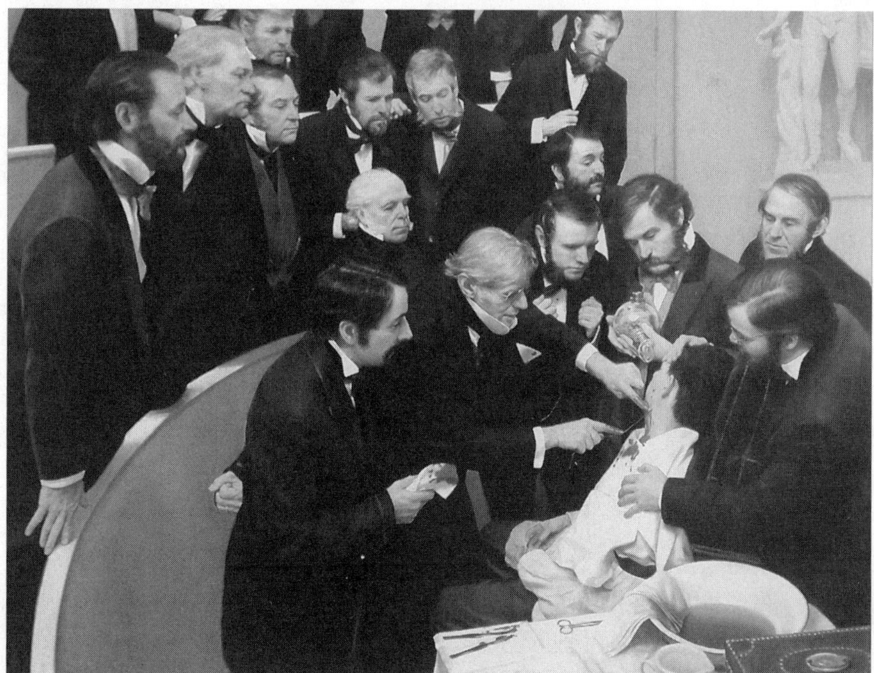

Figure 16: Depiction of event at Ether Dome. Painting by Warren and Lucia Prosperi, dated 2001. Courtesy of Massachusetts General Hospital Archives and Special Collections.

Warren anointed the discovery of surgical anesthesia as "the most valuable discovery ever made" with his enthusiastic statement:

> A new era has opened to the operating surgeon. His visitations on the most delicate parts are performed, not only without the agonizing screams he has been accustomed to hear, but sometimes with a state of perfect insensibility, and, occasionally, even with an expression of pleasure on the part of the patient. That is the most amazing miracle of all. Who could have imagined that drawing a knife over the delicate skin of the face might produce a sensation of unmixed delight? That the turning and twisting of instruments in the most sensitive parts might be accompanied by a delightful dream? If Ambroise Paré and Louis, and Dessault and Cheselden, Cooper and Hunter could see what our eyes daily witness, how would they long to come along with us and perform their exploits once more. It is the most valuable discovery ever made, because it frees suffering humanity from pain. Unrestrained and free as God's own sunshine it has gone forth to cheer and gladden the earth; it will awaken the gratitude of the present, and of all coming generations. The student who from distant lands or in distant ages, may visit this spot will view it with increased interest, as he remembers that here was first demonstrated one of the most glorious truths of science.[10]

Morton had grandiose schemes for the future. In keeping with his intention to apply for a patent for the process, he initially withheld the identity of ether, referring to the agent as "Letheon," from the river Lethe of Greek mythology, the water that erased painful memories. When news of the success spread, Horace Wells laid claim to the discovery of surgical anesthesia and even indicated that he had considered the use of sulphuric ether. After the magnitude of the discovery became appreciated, Charles Thomas Jackson made his allegedly seminal participation known.

Jackson (fig. 17), the most scientific of the three claimants, was a Harvard Medical School graduate as well as a noted chemist and geologist in Boston who had a tendency to confabulate and aggrandize the ideas of others. He tried to engage Alexis St. Martin, William Beaumont's subject, for his own studies. Jackson also claimed that he was the inventor of the electromagnetic telegraph and that he had given the idea to Samuel F. B. Morse during a sea voyage from Europe in October 1832. He also contested C. F. Schonbein's 1845 discovery of the explosive known as guncotton, claiming he was truly the discoverer. It is known, however, that Morton consulted with Jackson before the ether demonstration at Massachusetts General Hospital took place and that Jackson did suggest the use of sulphuric ether to Morton.

On November 21, 1846, Oliver Wendell Holmes, the poet, physician, and anatomist who became dean of Harvard Medical School, wrote to William Morton:

> Everybody wants to have a hand in a great discovery. All I will do is to give you a hint or two, as to names, or the name, to the state produced and the agent. . . . The state should, I think, be called "Anaesthesia." . . . The adjective will be "Anaesthetic." Thus we might say, the state of anaesthesia, or the anaesthetic state."[11]

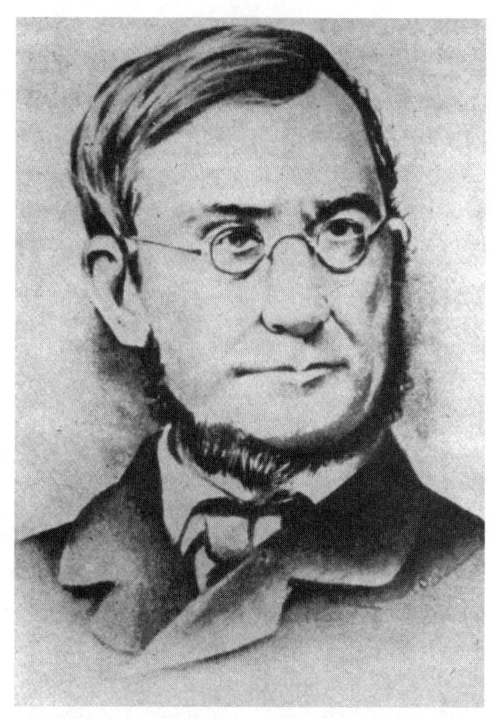

Figure 17: Charles Thomas Jackson. Courtesy Massachusetts General Hospital Archives and Special Collections.

The word "anaesthesia" was widely used at the time and dates to the first century when Dioscorides, a celebrated Greek physician, introduced it.

The first application for a patent on surgical anesthesia was taken out in the names of Morton and Jackson, whose inclusion was largely based on his scientific reputation rather than his contribution. Later, Jackson agreed to assign all his rights to Morton in exchange for 10 percent of all profits that accrued from American sales. Patent 4848 was issued by the United States Patent Office on November 12, 1846. The use of ether anesthesia rapidly spread around the world. On December 21, 1846, Robert Liston, England's most famous surgeon, performed the first operations, an amputation and the removal of a great toenail, under ether anesthesia at the University Hospital in London. Immediate British enthusiasm is evidenced by correspondence from a Dr. R. H. Collyer, who wrote:

> There should be public acts of thanksgiving throughout the land, for this signal favour to man and to come. Let young and old be earnest for this privilege, with their clergy, and let physicians and surgeons be the first to bow the knee.[12]

Surgeons in France, Germany, and Russia rapidly followed suit. The famous Russian surgeon Nikolai Ivanovich Pirigoff became one of the most vociferous champions of its use.

The widespread acceptance of ether as an agent to achieve surgical anesthesia was accompanied with even more efforts by the claimants for recognition of priority. When Horace Wells, William T. G. Morton, and Charles T. Jackson individually came to an appreciation of the potential for the discovery, each staked his claim. In December 1846, Wells had a letter published in the *Hartford Courant* that first stated his case. While in Paris on nonmedical business, he sent his claim for priority to the Académie des Sciences in February 1847. Jackson had previously written a letter, dated November 13, 1846, for submission to the Académie des Sciences claiming that he was the sole discoverer of the anesthetic use of sulphuric ether and that he was responsible for its introduction into surgical practice by his agent, a "dentist of this city." After over three years of deliberation, the Académie des Sciences determined that the Montyon Prize, and the title "Benefactor of Mankind," was to be shared by Wells and Jackson.

The ensuing lives of the three men, who had staked their respective claims to be the original discoverer of surgical anesthesia, were characterized by extreme tragedy. Horace Wells's failure to achieve what he deemed to be appropriate recognition led to an intense depression and addiction to drugs and chloroform—curiously, the latter followed ether as an agent for inhalation anesthesia. He was jailed in New York City for throwing sulfuric acid at a prostitute. In jail, he committed suicide by slashing his femoral artery with a razor. Charles T. Jackson died at age seventy-five, in 1880, having spent the last seven years of his life in a mental institution.

William T. G. Morton received the most recognition for the discovery of surgical anesthesia. His honors included a gold medal from the Académie des Sciences, the Cross of the Order of St. Vladimir from the Tsar of All the Russias, the Cross of the Order of Vasa from the king of Sweden, and election in 1920 to the famous New York University Hall of Fame. Despite all this recognition, his patent was not sustained and his three petitions to Congress for compensation failed. He attempted farming, only to progress to a state of squalor and poverty. He died a disappointed man in New York City in 1868 following a stroke. Of the three claimants, however, Morton is regarded as the most deserving of accolades. A monument was erected over his grave at the Mount Auburn cemetery in Boston. The inscription reads:

> INVENTOR AND REVEALER OF ANAESTHETIC INHALATION BY WHOM, PAIN IN SURGERY WAS ARRESTED AND ANNULLED BEFORE WHOM, IN ALL TIME, SURGERY WAS AGONY SINCE WHOM, SCIENCE HAS CONTROL OF PAIN.

On the fiftieth anniversary of the first public demonstration of surgical anesthesia, S. Weir Mitchell, the famous physician, author, and poet, produced a commemorative poem for the occasion. In the verse he extolled the contribution of William Thomas Green Morton with the lines:

> How did we thank him? Ah! No joy-bells ring
> No pæans greeted, and no poets sang;
> No cannons thundered from the guarded strand
> This mighty victory to a grateful land!
> We took the gift so humbly, simply given,
> And, coldly selfish—left out debt to Heaven.
> How shall we thank him? Hush! A gladder hour
> Has struck to him; a wiser, juster power
> Shall know full well how fitly to reward
> The generous soul that found the world so hard.[13]

In assessing the value of surgical anesthesia, Mitchell wrote:

> Whatever triumphs still shall hold the mind.
> Whatever gift shall yet enrich mankind,
> Ah! Here, no hour shall strike through all the years,
> No hour as sweet, as when hope, doubt and fears,
> Mid-deepening stillness, watched on eager brain,
> With God-like will, decree the Death of Pain.[14]

CHAPTER 6:

TWO PRIME TARGETS

Surgery does the ideal thing—it separates the patient from his disease. It puts the patient back to bed and the disease in a bottle.

—Logan Clendening
Modern Methods of Treatment (1924)

According to the United States national database, as reported on a government Web site, approximately 430,000 gallbladders and 330,000 appendixes were removed in 2003. Discounting gynecologic operations, removal of the gallbladder and the appendix constituted the most commonly performed intra-abdominal procedures. Thus, in recent years, they have been the general surgeon's two prime targets.

During the second half of the nineteenth century, European medicine and surgery continued to enjoy a position of world leadership while the United States was still evolving both medically and scientifically. American surgeons did, however, make seminal contributions to the treatment of the diseased gallbladder and appendix. In the time before these American contributions to surgery were made, the domestic strife that culminated in the Civil War limited the potential for medical advancement within the United States. Nonetheless, wars characteristically have generated surgical innovations. During the War between the States, the use of an improved ambulance corps, patterned after the one initiated by Baron Larrey during the Napoleonic campaigns, had a significant impact on mortality rates. The word "band-aid" memorializes the evacuation vehicles that were manned by members of the regimental bands.

The other medical advance that occurred during the Civil War was that, for the first time in history, data were collected and analyzed for mortality and morbidity during a conflict. Deaths due to injuries and illnesses were quantified as were the types of amputations and wound treatments performed. The surgeon general's office of the time, the repository for this information, can be regarded as the precursor to the complex bastions of medical information now included in the missions of the National Institutes of Health, the National Medical Library, and the Centers for Disease Control and Prevention.

After the internecine conflict ended, an unprecedented and, for a long-time, unduplicated surgical experience took place in yet another improbable locale. For the first time, on June 15, 1867, a successful operation was performed on a patient's gallbladder. The improbable location was the third floor of a wholesale drug company in Indianapolis, Indiana, miles from the established East Coast medical centers. The operator was a fifty-seven-year-old surgeon by the name of John Stough Bobbs.

John Stough Bobbs (fig. 18) was born in Green Village, Pennsylvania, in 1809, the same year as Abraham Lincoln, Charles Darwin, and Oliver Wendell Holmes. That year also witnessed Ephraim McDowell's elective operation within the abdominal cavity. Bobbs, like McDowell, Beaumont, and Sims, followed the practice of the time by initiating his medical education as an apprentice to a local physician. He began his studies with Dr. Martin Luther in Harrisburg, Pennsylvania, before proceeding in 1835 to Jefferson Medical College, which also had educated Ephraim McDowell, and J. Marion Sims. Bobbs, however, did not complete the studies required to receive a doctor of medicine degree at that institution.

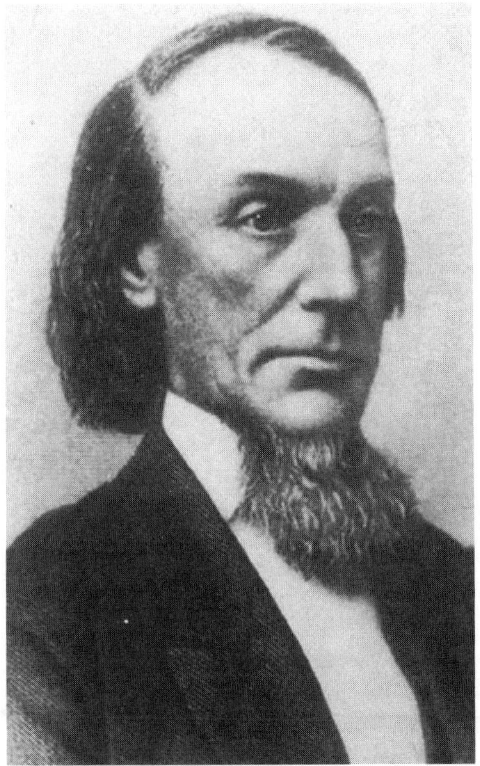

Figure 18: John Stough Bobbs. Courtesy of Indiana State Medical Society.

This lack of a degree did not preclude him from playing major roles in the medical organizations and medical educational institutes in Indianapolis, where he began to practice before he had left for Jefferson Medical College. He was a founder and the first secretary of the Indianapolis Medical Society, and he organized the formation of the Indiana State Medical Society. In 1849, when the Indiana Central Medical School was established in Indianapolis under the aegis of Asbury College, which later became DePauw University, John Stough Bobbs was designated the first dean, and also served as professor of anatomy and surgery. His broader influence in the state is evidenced by four years of service as a state senator.

During the Civil War, Bobbs maintained his civilian status, but he actively participated in medical matters related to the Union Army. He took part in the first military campaign in Virginia and later served as chief surgeon for General George McClelland in the southern theater. Toward the end of the conflict, Bobbs was medical director for the district of Indiana and cared for prisoners of war in an Indianapolis detention camp.

The significant surgical event in which Bobbs was the active participant took place in 1867 in Indianapolis, which at the time was a modest city with a population of about forty-five thousand. Coincidentally, that year was also marked by the Scottish surgeon Joseph Lister's revolutionary reports that introduced aseptic (free from disease germs) surgery.

On June 15, a local seamstress referred to as "E. W." (later identified as Mary E. Wiggins) underwent an operative procedure by Bobbs at her own insistence in spite of his initial reluctance. For years, she had experienced abdominal symptoms that were initially attributed to an ovarian tumor. When she could no longer cope with the discomfort, and when the mass had expanded to a size that interfered with her ability to work, she sought Bobbs's assistance. Although he did not appreciate the nature of the tumor preoperatively, Bobbs thought that it was unlikely to be of ovarian origin.

The operation took place on the third floor of Kiefer's and Vinton's Wholesale Drug Company at 26 South Meridian Street, Indianapolis, because, in the absence of a fully equipped operating room and recovery room in a hospital in the region, the space in the drug company provided a convenient venue. One advantage was that Bobbs's office was located at 18 E. Washington Street, only a short distance away in a building now occupied by the State Life Insurance Company.

The operation was performed under anesthesia induced by chloroform, an agent that had been discovered in 1831 almost simultaneously by Samuel Guthrie in the United States and by Eugene Souberian in France, and later popularized as an anesthetic agent by James Simpson of England in 1847, one year after ether was first administered to achieve surgical anesthesia. Five local physicians and a medical student assisted Bobbs in the operation.

The abdominal cavity was entered directly over the palpable mass through a right paramedian vertical incision that extended from above the navel to the pubic area. This is the same incision that would still be used by some surgeons when the nature of an abdominal mass could not be defined preoperatively. Once the tumor was visualized and examined directly, it was noted to have an oval shape and to be five inches long and two inches wide. There was a broad connection to the liver, and, therefore, the tumor could not be removed from the wound.

Because the tumor obviously contained liquid contents, an incision was made that resulted in the forceful expulsion of fluid and several pellet-sized masses. Bobbs introduced his finger into the cystic mass and removed several individual, solid pebblelike objects of varying sizes. One small hard mass was found at what was probably the junction of the gallbladder and the cystic duct, but it could not be removed. Bobbs explains in his published description of the operation:

> No pedicle could be made out, and the sack showing its contents to be transparent, its lower margin was cut through, when a perfectly limpid fluid escaped, propelling, with considerable force, several solid bodies about the size of ordinary rifle bullets. Introducing the finger other solid bodies were felt, but not in the main sack. A number were hooked out with the finger, and varied in size from that of a mustard seed to that of a bullet. One of the latter sized could be distinctly felt, but no communication between the space containing this and the main sack could be found, and it was not removed, being at the extreme end of the finger.[1]

Once it was determined that the fluid-filled mass was broadly attached to the lower surface of the right lobe of the liver, Bobbs deduced that he had probably evacuated a distended gallbladder. The extent of the attachment deterred removal of the cystic mass and the opening was closed with a suture, bringing together the cut edges to prevent spillage of the solid contents into the abdominal cavity and also to encourage the formation of adhesions between the sac's surface and the inner (peritoneal) surface of the abdominal wall. Fusion of the sac's surface and the abdominal wall would facilitate the insertion of a trochar (rigid tube) for evacuation in the event of reaccumulation of fluid within the cystic mass. The abdominal wound was closed with sutures and a dressing was applied.

Medical knowledge regarding the gallbladder and its diseases, including stones, was limited at the time of Bobbs's operation. The ancient Greeks were curiously silent about gallstones. It was the Roman Tralianus, in the sixth century, who first made definite mention of gallstones within the hepatic ducts. In the sixteenth century, both Andreas Vesalius and his pupil Gabrielle Fallopius described stones within the gallbladders of dissected bodies. Also during that century, Antonio Benevieni of Florence and Jean Fernel, physician to the king of France, presented the earliest accounts of correlations between clinical manifestations and the presence of gallstones. In 1618, Farbricius Hildanus (William Fabry), the Father of German Surgery, in Bern, Switzerland, removed a gallstone from a living patient.

In 1733, Jean Louis Petit first suggested that a large inflamed gallbladder that was firmly adherent to the abdominal wall necessitated drainage and removal of the calculi, or stones. Ten years later he successfully performed the procedure without entering the general abdominal cavity. In 1859, the German chemist T. L. W. Thudichum suggested that the diseased gallbladder should be marsupialized, permanently exposing the inside of the gallbladder to the skin, so that stones could be removed later without violating the abdominal cavity.

The operation performed by Bobbs should have been designated as a "cholecystostomy" rather than the incorrect term, "cholecystotomy," which he used because the former indicates opening and closure, while the latter defines the creation of a persistent opening. Analysis of the operative procedure in the light of modern standards of practice would evoke loud and almost universal criticism. It is inappropriate to close a diseased distended gallbladder, particularly when the operating surgeon is cognizant of having left behind an impacted stone. Recurrence or continuance of the disease process with reaccumulation of fluid within the gallbladder and infection of the fluid within a closed space would be anticipated, resulting in the return of the original symptoms, pain, and probable dire consequences, perhaps leading to death.

The modern experts would be surprised to learn that, in the case of Mary E. Wiggins, they would have been wrong. The patient had a relatively uneventful recovery. She sat up two weeks after the operation, walked in three weeks, and left her place of care in four weeks, a time pattern consistent with that associated with other surgical procedures in the mid-nineteenth century. During a ten-month period of follow-up, she experienced intermittent fevers and indigestion, but was ultimately able to return to work.

The patient married sometime subsequent to the operation. In 1905, she was exhibited to an audience of physicians at a meeting of the American Medical Association in Portland, Oregon. She lived to the age of seventy-seven, forty-six years following her procedure with only occasional episodes of abdominal discomfort. The scenario followed the pattern of Dr. Ephraim McDowell and Jane Todd Crawford, Dr. William Beaumont and Alexis St. Martin, and Dr. J. Marion Sims and Anarcha in that the patient once again outlived the surgeon.

One year after the momentous operation, Bobbs became the nineteenth president of the Indiana State Medical Society. In that capacity, he urged that a state medical school and a state medical journal should be established. At his inaugural address, he read a paper titled "Case of Lithotomy of the Gall Bladder," which included another misnomer in terminology—"lithotomy," which actually means cutting *of* a stone rather than *for* a stone. The paper was published in 1868, in volume 18 of the *Transactions of the Indiana State Medical Society*, a journal with a limited and geographically confined circulation. The medical world, in general, was uninformed of the event.

In 1869, the Indiana Medical College was established and John Stough Bobbs was appointed president of the faculty and professor of surgery. Exactly six months to the day after the school was opened, Bobbs died of a respiratory infection. All the local obituaries failed to mention the seminal operation that he had performed. Even the tributes in the state medical journal, including one written by a physician who was present at the procedure, neglected to note his unique surgical contribution. Recognition of Bobbs's innovative operation would be delayed for twelve years.

No surgeon operated on the gallbladder for eleven years subsequent to Bobbs's experience. J. Marion Sims performed the next operation on the gallbladder on an American woman in Paris in 1878. At the time, Sims was unaware of Bobbs's accomplishment. In Sims's case, he opened a distended gallbladder, removed about sixty stones, and sewed the edges of the gallbladder opening to the wound in order to allow for persistent drainage. Postoperatively, the patient developed diffuse bleeding from several sites and died eight days after the operation.

Sims was unacquainted with Bobbs's publication as evidenced by his statement: "I believe this operation is unique. . . . As this operation is new we must find a name for it."[2] Sims suggested "cholecystotomy." The correct term would be "cholecystostomy" because a persistent opening was created. This procedure remains in the current surgical armamentarium as an infrequently performed operation for a very ill patient who is considered to be unable to tolerate removal of the diseased organ.

Two months after Sims's operation, Theodor Kocher of Bern, Switzerland, who in 1909 would become the first surgeon to receive the Nobel Prize in Physiology or Medicine for his contribution to an understanding of "the physiology, pathology, and surgery of diseases of the thyroid gland," successfully performed a two-staged procedure on the gallbladder. He first sewed the gallbladder to the wall of the abdomen and, at a later date, established external drainage. He made no mention of Bobbs's experience.

Also in 1878, W. W. Keen of Philadelphia performed a cholecystostomy for empyema (purulence, or a pussy discharge) of the gallbladder in a sixty-year-old woman, who died thirty-six hours after the operation. Once again, the surgeon failed to recognize Bobbs's accomplishment and, instead, referred to Sims's operation that had been reported in the widely read *British Medical Journal* of June 8, 1878, as the only previous procedure.

Drainage of the diseased gallbladder entered the category of acceptable surgical procedures as a consequence of the successes achieved by Lawson Tait, the distinguished English surgeon from Birmingham. He reported his first successful drainage with removal of two large gallstones from a distended gallbladder in the *Lancet* in 1879.[3] Over half of the first twenty-seven documented cases of drainage were performed by Tait, who also referred to Sims's experience and failed to mention Bobbs.

In the same year that Tait's first report appeared, Bobbs was finally credited with the first successful operation on the gallbladder. However, the article attesting to Bobbs's primacy appeared in the same obscure journal that published Bobbs's original paper.[4] As the nineteenth century was drawing to a close, thirty-one years after the fact, the editor of the *Indiana State Medical Journal* reproduced Bobbs's original article and mailed copies to many notable surgeons in the United States.[5] Bobbs's contribution was finally acknowledged throughout the world.

John Stough Bobbs is memorialized on the wall of the Indiana Public Library by a bronze plaque bearing a relief image of his likeness and two succinct statements: "Illustrious Surgeon, Patriotic Citizen, Self-Sacrificing

Benefactor, Servant of God through Service to Mankind," and "First to Perform the Operation of Cholecystotomy."

The first successful elective removal of the gallbladder was performed at the Lazarus Hospital in Berlin in July 1882 by Carl Langenbuch. Langenbuch conducted animal experiments before embarking on the procedure and stated that "the gallbladder should be removed not because it contains stones, but because it forms them," emphasizing that the organ is diseased in these cases. Throughout the remainder of the nineteenth century and the early part of the twentieth century, European surgeons dominated the field of surgery on the gallbladder and biliary tract.

Finally, in 1987, with the introduction of laparoscopic removal of the gallbladder by Erich Mühe in Germany and its popularization by François Dubois and Philippe Mouret in France, cholecystectomy underwent a dramatic change. The ability to remove the diseased organ by using three small abdominal ports to allow for visualization, magnification, dissection, and excision instead of a larger abdominal incision resulted in reduced hospital stay and earlier return to normal activity. Minimally invasive surgery contributed to a more liberal application of the procedure that was elevated to the number one position on the list of frequently performed intra-abdominal operations, exclusive of those directed at gynecologic organs.

John Stough Bobbs's operation on the gallbladder was seminal but had no influence in the surgical world and therefore might readily be discounted. On the other hand, invoking the statement of Jonathan Swift: "He was a bold man that first ate an oyster." Bobbs's contribution certainly merits the accolade of "Boldness!"

In contrast to the lack of initial recognition for an American surgeon's first successful operation on the gallbladder, America's contribution to the understanding of appendicitis and removal of the appendix was immediately influential in changing medical and surgical attitudes around the world. This significant American contribution to surgery came not from a surgeon but rather from a pathologist.

The need to remove the vermiform (wormlike) appendix ranks second in frequency of intra-abdominal organs, exclusive of the uterus and ovaries. It is exceeded only by the gallbladder. For an organ that can be classified as vestigial, it certainly has evoked surgical interest out of proportion to its size and function.

There is evidence that the Egyptians had knowledge of the organ because in the process of mummification the abdominal viscera were removed and placed in Coptic jars with some bearing inscriptions referring to the "worm" of the intestine. But, in the times of Greek and Roman medicine, related to the influence of Celsus and Galen in the first and second centuries CE, respectively, the appendix was not identified, because dissections were limited to animals without an appendix.

Ignorance of the existence of the appendix persisted throughout the Middle Ages, and its identification represents the increasing interest in human anatomy that evolved during the Renaissance. The small, usually inconsequential part of the gastrointestinal tract was depicted in an anatomic drawing by Leonardo da Vinci, who began performing his anatomic studies in Milan in the 1480s. In about 1492, Leonardo drew the appendix as a distinct offshoot of the cecum (the first portion of the large intestine) and assigned it the name "orrechio," meaning ear. His description, however, had little impact because his anatomic drawings were not published until the nineteenth century.

The appendix was first depicted in print by Andreas Vesalius, the Belgian anatomist who taught at the University of Padua in Italy. The representation appeared in the fifth volume of the classic *De Humani Corporis Fabrica* (1543). As was true of all of Vesalius's illustrations, it was based on his dissection of a human cadaver. Vesalius assigned the name "caecum," meaning blind pouch, to the appendix itself. The current name evolved in 1710 when Philip Verheyen, the Dutch surgeon who is associated with the phenomenon that is now referred to as the "Phantom Limb," applied the term "appendix vermiformis."

Some historians ascribe the first description of appendicitis to Jean Fernel, who noted and reported a perforated appendix during an autopsy of a seven-year-old girl in 1544. In 1767, the great English surgeon John Hunter identified a gangrenous appendix at an autopsy. During the first half of the eighteenth century, several Parisian physicians, based on their recognition of gangrenous appendixes at autopsy, suggested removing the organ in patients who had symptoms suggestive of peritonitis. But Baron Guillaume Dupuytren, the most influential French surgeon of his time, squelched the suggestion. Instead he indicted "typhlitis," an inflammatory process of the cecum, as the cause of the symptoms and pathology. In the 1830s, two English physicians, Richard Bright and Thomas Addison, whose names are attached to nephritis and adrenal insufficiency, respectively, described the symptom complex of appendicitis and implicated the appendix itself in their text *Elements of the Practice of Medicine* (1839). They indicated that appendicitis was the most frequent cause of inflammation in the right lower quadrant of the abdomen, but removal was not considered. James Copeland, in his *Dictionary of Practical Medicine* (1836), was the first to discriminate between inflammation of the cecum and that of the appendix.

The first chronicled appendectomy took place on December 6, 1735, when Claudius Amyand, sergeant surgeon to King George II of Great Britain, operated on an eleven-year-old boy at St. George's Hospital in London for a hernia that had extended into the scrotum and was draining intestinal contents through the skin. When the hernia sac was opened, it was noted that a pin perforated the appendix. The appendix was removed, the fistula closed, and the patient recovered. The case was recorded in the *Philosophical Transactions of the Royal Society* in 1736.[6]

The next appendectomy in Great Britain occurred after a hiatus of 145 years when Lawson Tait, the nation's leading surgeon who played a significant role in operations on the gallbladder, diagnosed appendicitis with rupture in a seventeen-year-old female and successfully removed it. The case, however, was not reported for ten years, by which time Tait personally had abandoned the procedure.

In keeping with the pattern established for American surgery throughout the nineteenth century, technical advancements and bold incursions related to the appendix were products of surgeons distant from the East Coast urban centers. Abraham Groves performed the first elective appendectomy for nonruptured acute appendicitis diagnosed preoperatively in 1883 on a twelve-year-old boy in the small community of Fergus, Ontario, Canada. The case was not reported until it appeared in Groves's autobiography in 1934.[7] The first successful appendectomy in the United States was performed by William West Grant in Davenport, Iowa, in 1885. Once again, the case was not reported at the time and didn't appear until 1933.[8]

America's significant contribution to the worldwide appreciation of acute appendicitis took place at the inaugural meeting of the Association of American Physicians in Washington, DC, in June 1886. The contribution was made by Reginald H. Fitz (fig. 19), Shattuck Professor of Pathology at Harvard

Medical School. In an extensive twenty-eight-page article, Fitz suggested that the term "appendicitis" should be applied, replacing "typhlitis" and "perityphlitis," which were considered to be vague and inappropriate in focusing attention on an inflammatory process in the cecum. He described in detailed and deliberate terms the symptoms and signs of the disease and the potential course of the pathologic process as it moves from local inflammation to gangrene and perforation, diffuse peritonitis or abscess formation. Fitz concluded that it is essential to diagnose the disease early; in most instances the diagnosis is easy, and exploration of the abdomen should be performed early at which time the appendix should be removed.[9]

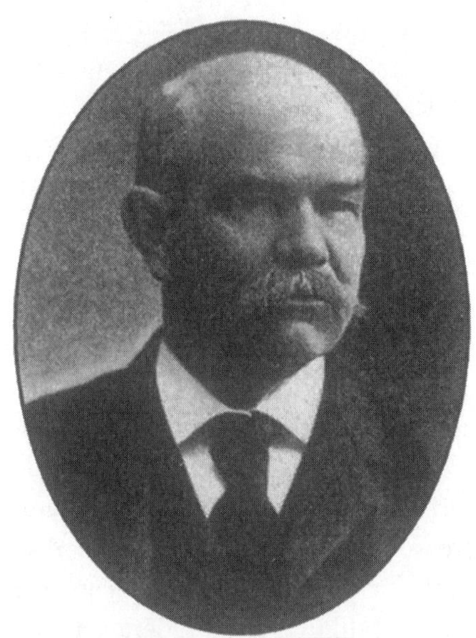

Figure 19: Reginald H. Fitz. Courtesy of Massachusetts General Hospital Archives and Special Collections.

Reginald Fitz's evangelical message was immediately taken up with apostolic zeal by two prominent American surgeons, Charles McBurney of New York City and John B. Murphy of Chicago. McBurney published a series of papers that advised early intervention whereupon his name was forever affixed to the point of maximal tenderness in the right lower quadrant of the abdomen, "located exactly between an inch and a half and two inches from the anterior spinous process of the ileum on a straight line from that process to the umbilicus."[10] His name is also assigned to an incision that is often employed to remove the appendix.

In Chicago there were two therapeutic encampments related to the treatment of appendicitis and peritonitis. Albert J. Ochsner of Chicago advocated nonoperative treatment for peritonitis caused by appendicitis, in other words, delaying an operation until an abscess was established at which point drainage was performed.[11] By contrast, in the same city, John B. Murphy championed early and rapid operation. In 1904, he reported on two thousand appendectomies he had personally performed.[12] The focal point of criticism by colleagues and adulation by patients, Murphy was charismatic and bigger than life, as evidenced by the monumental, pillared auditorium that stands as a memorial to him on Erie Street, just a block from the Miracle Mile of Chicago.

George R. Fowler of the Polyclinic Graduate School in New York City, the first postgraduate medical institution in the United States, also contributed significantly to our knowledge of appendicitis. In 1894, he published the first textbook that focused on appendicitis, and his name has been attached to the semisitting position that was used to encourage the localization of an abscess associated with peritonitis to the pelvis.[13] Coincidentally, he died due to peritonitis following an operation on a perforated appendix.

Unlike the usual circumstance during the end of the nineteenth and the early twentieth century in which surgical concepts and operative innovations crossed the Atlantic Ocean in a westerly direction, the reverse was true for appendicitis. One of the first surgeons in Great Britain to adopt the precepts of Reginald Fitz was Frederick Treves, whose daughter died from complications of acute appendicitis without undergoing an operation. Within months of Fitz's publication in the *American Journal of Medical Sciences*, Treves operated on a patient for symptoms attributed to the appendix. The operation consisted of straightening the appendix rather than removal of the organ, the former being an operative procedure that is never justified. The patient recovered uneventfully.

Treves's most notable patient with a diseased appendix was King Edward VII, who, on the eve of his scheduled coronation, was evaluated for abdominal pain of ten days' duration. The condition worsened, requiring drainage of an appendiceal abscess at Buckingham Palace and delay of the coronation. The king recovered and lived for another eight years; Treves was made a baronet. Shortly thereafter, Treves gave up surgery to write a series of widely read travel books and is now best remembered as the author of *The Elephant Man and Other Reminiscences.*

During the final decade of the twentieth century, advancement in surgical techniques resulted in the diseased appendix joining the diseased gallbladder as an organ more frequently removed by laparoscopic surgery. Appendectomy assumed second place on the list of frequency for nongynecologic abdominal organs removed through this approach.

CHAPTER 7:

TWO OFT-FORGOTTEN CONTRIBUTIONS

Instruction in medicine is like the culture of the Earth. For our natural disposition is, as it were, the soil; the tenets of our teacher are, as it were, the seed; instruction in youth is like planting of the seed in the ground at the proper season; the place where the instruction is communicated is like the food imparted to the vegetables by the atmosphere; diligent study is like the cultivation of the fields; and it is time which imparts strength to all things and brings them to maturity.

—Hippocrates (ca. 450 BCE)

Johns Hopkins Hospital was the focal point for two revolutionary contributions that continue to have an impact on the discipline of surgery. Although the two American surgeons responsible for these contributions were each highly regarded for their surgical prowess, one surgeon's contribution was of a broader dimension that extended beyond both the medical and the surgical professions and into society. Similarly, the most lasting contributions of the second surgeon have transcended the operating theater in which his reputation was established.

The first surgeon, John Shaw Billings, was responsible for both collating and facilitating the acquisition of all aspects of medical information. The second surgeon, William Stewart Halsted, revolutionized surgical training. The former developed the plans for Johns Hopkins Hospital while the latter used the same hospital as the arena for his activities. Together, the two men arguably deserve the most significant credit for raising the standard of American surgery to its position of worldwide leadership. While Billings "did more to advance the status of American Medicine than any other man of his time," Halsted was America's best-known surgeon during the end of the nine-

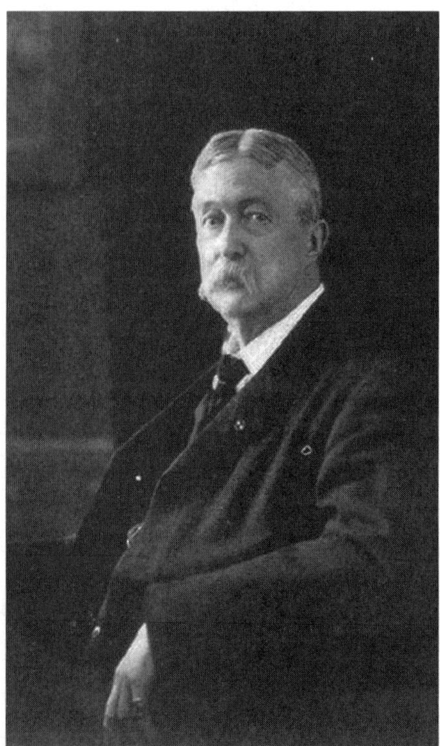

Figure 20: John Shaw Billings. Courtesy of the Alan Mason Chesney Medical Archives, Johns Hopkins Medical Institutions, photograph by Rockwood, Baltimore, Maryland.

teenth century and the early part of the twentieth century.[1] In conjunction, their contributions to American medicine and surgery were of immense proportions.

John Shaw Billings (fig. 20) was born on April 12, 1838, in Cotton Township, Indiana. In 1860, after graduating from Miami University of Ohio, he went on to receive his medical degree at the Medical College of Ohio (Cincinnati), the tenth-oldest medical school in the nation and the second oldest, following Transylvania University in Lexington, Kentucky, west of the Allegheny Mountains. Upon graduation, he became demonstrator of anatomy at the Medical College of Ohio and participated in the surgical practice of Professor George C. Blackman until the outbreak of the Civil War.

In 1862, Billings accepted an appointment as first lieutenant and assistant surgeon in the medical corps of the United States Army and became one of "those young men of 1861 who laid their professional gifts on the military altar."[2] By May 1862 Billings took charge of Cliffburne Hospital, a sprawling tented encampment on a hill behind Georgetown in Washington, DC, which the United States Fifth Cavalry had previously occupied. It was there that Billings first instituted sanitary reforms and had the "opportunity to acquire a reputation and surgical glory."[3]

After a six-month tour as executive officer of the large United States Army General Hospital in west Philadelphia, where his administrative activities and complex surgical operations occupied long hours, Billings left his desk for the battlefield. Billings exhibited his surgical skills at the battles of

Chancellorsville (May 1–3, 1863) and Gettysburg (July 1–3, 1863). His new position, however, was not without its risk; at Chancellorsville Billings replaced a surgeon who had been killed and one of his assistants was also killed. During Gettysburg, Billings was in charge of the field hospital of the Second Division of the Fifth Corps, where he performed numerous and diverse operations on the extremities, torso, and cranium and "had [his] left ear just touched with a ball."[4]

From October 1863 through March 1864, Billings was stationed at hospital facilities on islands in New York Harbor and then, at his own request, was transferred to the Army of the Potomac around Washington, DC, where he served as a medical inspector. Billings participated in the battle of the Wilderness (May 5–6, 1864) and the Army of the Potomac's ensuing battles until the end of July when he was granted a leave. Billings was regarded as one of the ablest surgeons on the battlefield and is credited with being the first surgeon in the war to successfully remove the ankle joint—a procedure that, according to published reports, had only been performed on two or three previous occasions. While serving with the Army of the Potomac, Billings also coordinated the ambulances on the battlefields, the care of the patients who were triaged to medical facilities, along with the first organized attempt to collect statistical data regarding injuries, operations, medical illnesses, and pathologic specimens during warfare. The responsibility of coordinating these efforts provided Billings with invaluable experience for his future endeavors.

Due to the recognition of his administrative talents, Billings was assigned for a short period to the office of the medical director in Washington, DC. At the end of 1864, he took up a post at the Surgeon General's Office, where he would remain until his retirement thirty years later. It was there, amid days of drudgery, that his genius would manifest and his reputation would soar. He would generate two contributions that continue to affect the acquisition and dissemination of surgical and medical knowledge to this day.

Billings's initial focus on routine office management and the supervision of clerks conducting bookkeeping and fiscal affairs furthered his administrative skills. It also allowed him the time to develop a proficiency in microscopy, which would become applicable during his subsequent bacteriologic studies associated with hygiene. Around 1870, Billings received two specific assignments that would transform his career and lead to his ultimate position of expertise and dominance in the disparate realms of bibliography, hygiene, and the organization and management of hospitals.

Billings was charged with conducting an in-depth analysis of the Marine Hospital Service that was responsible for the care of disabled sailors and the Quarantine Service that manned ports of entry into the country. His reports to the surgeon general, "Barracks and Hospitals" and "The Hygiene of the United States Army," were replete with criticisms and stimulated significant modifications regarding medical facilities and protocols. The reports remained pertinent historic references for many years and also served as a starting point for the eventual formation in 1912 of the Public Health Service. Billings also became active in the American Public Health Association and was elected to its presidency in 1880. That association was central to the initiation and performance of a systematic survey of the status of sanitation in the United States.

Between 1875 and 1876, as the nation prepared for its centennial celebrations, Billings exhibited his bibliographic expertise in three major works. The first, the *Bibliography of Cholera* (1875), provided a presentation of the complete literature on the subject to date. The second, *Specimen Fasiculus of a Catalogue of the Medical Library, under the Direction of the Surgeon General, United States Army* (1877), was published as a trial balloon for his third major work, the *Index Catalogue* (1880), which was a complete compilation of the holdings of the Surgeon General's Library.

At the time of *Specimen Fasiculus*'s publication, the Surgeon General's Library contained about forty thousand volumes and an equal number of pamphlets. Because *Specimen Fasiculus* documented this vast collection, it was well received. Oliver Wendell Holmes, in his dedicatory address at the opening of the Boston Medical Hospital, singled out that work for praise and championed appropriation by Congress for expansion of the concept.[5]

During this same year of extraordinary productivity, Billings also completed *A Century of American Medicine, 1776–1876* (1876). In this book he expressed the opinion that the medical literature produced by colonial physicians was of little consequence. He regarded the only medical book published in America at the onset of the American Revolution—the one authored by Dr. John Jones in 1776, which focused on the treatment of wounds and fractures (see chapter 1)—as purely derivative, with the single exception of the observation that herniation of the brain occurred after creating a burr hole in the skull. Two contributions that did merit Billings's designation as significant were William Beaumont's experiments concerning digestion and the introduction of ether anesthesia (see chapters 2 and 5).

Billings's historical essay concludes with a succinct assessment of the status of medicine at the one hundredth anniversary of the nation. It speaks to the paucity of individuals who were truly interested in scientific inquiry and advancement. According to Billings, most physicians regarded the profession as a mechanism for gaining wealth, power, and social recognition. He also indicated that a large class of practicing physicians had been subjected to a deplorable medical education. Billings's report emphasized the need for extensive reforms in medical education, including standardization for admission, curriculum, and graduation at medical schools. This presaged the Flexner Report that was issued by the Carnegie Foundation for the Advancement of Teaching thirty-four years later and resulted in a revolutionary improvement in American medical education.

In 1873, a Baltimore merchant and banker named Johns Hopkins announced his grant of thirteen acres in Baltimore and a gift of $2 million in real estate, the revenue from which would be dedicated to the construction of a hospital. It was specified that the facility should concentrate on the care of indigents but should also allow for a limited number of paying patients.

Setting the tone that would persist through the years, the donor specifically insisted that the medical and surgical staff should be of the highest caliber and that the hospital should become an integral part of a concomitantly established university where the faculty would emphasize research and education. Thus, the flagship and standard for the future of medical education in the United States was established because the grant stated that the building should "provide for a hospital which shall, in structure and arrangement compare favorably with any other institution of like character in this country or in Europe."[6] This grant would also become a model for the goals of the subsequent Flexner Report.

Of the five building proposals that were submitted for the hospital in 1875, it was Billings's plan that was selected. Some of the specifics that contributed to the selection of his proposal were a two-story complex of buildings that incorporated administration under a single head, the inclusion of pathological and physiological laboratories, an out-patient facility, a nursing school, pharmacies, and a sophisticated system of records for the accumulation and maintenance of both medical and financial information on all patients.

Although Billings focused on such specifics as the heating and ventilation of the hospital buildings, he also emphasized that the most important element was the recruitment of a dynamic faculty of original investigators to guide the development of the institution. The buildings were to serve as an optimal environment for the faculty, students, and patients. Billings strongly opposed didactic clinical lectures and he especially opposed placing the patient on exhibition to students in an amphitheater. Instead, rather than learning through lecture and textbooks, education was to be based mainly on the observation of patients at their bedside and through practical experimentation.

On May 7, 1889, the Johns Hopkins Hospital (fig. 21), consisting of seventeen buildings surfaced with red bricks, formally opened. Before the structure was complete, however, in keeping with his emphasis on the essential element of an outstanding faculty, Billings played a major role in the 1884 selection of Professor William H. Welch as chair of pathology, the institution's first appointee and early dominant force. Billings also played a role in the 1888 recruitment of William Osler as the hospital's physician-in-chief.

Currently, *U. S. News & World Report* presents an annual list of the best hospitals in the United States. For fifteen consecutive years—from 1993 to

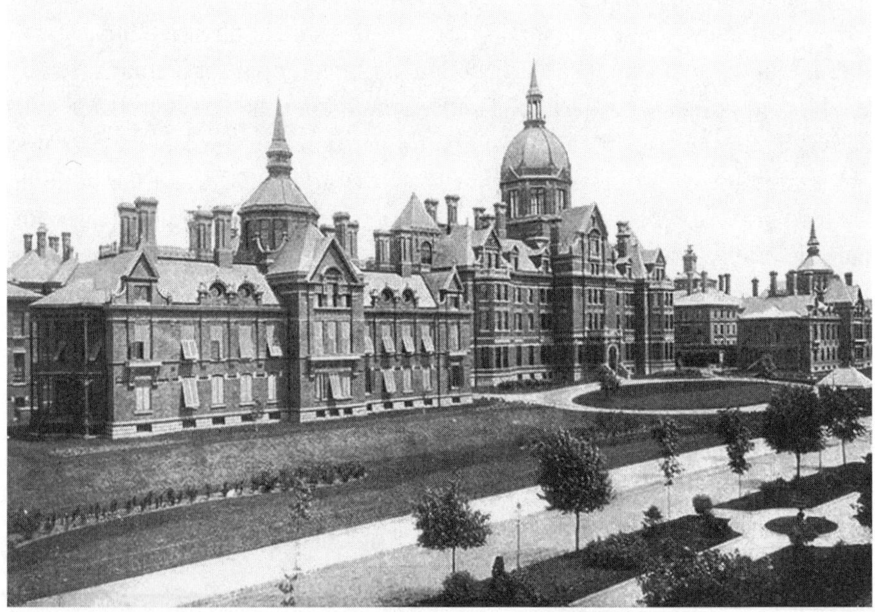

Figure 21: Johns Hopkins Hospital at the time of completion. Courtesy of the Alan Mason Chesney Archives, Johns Hopkins Medical Institutions. Photograph by Gutenkunst, Baltimore, Maryland.

2008—Johns Hopkins Hospital, the distinguished institution that Billings was the dominant force in planning and establishing, has headed the list. Billings's expertise in the realm of hospital planning was once again called upon in 1905 to lay out plans for the proposed Peter Bent Brigham Hospital in Boston.

As impressive as John Shaw Billings was as the creator of great hospitals, his most significant contribution to all of medicine is the bibliographic system that he developed while serving as the director of the Surgeon General's Library. Between 1865 and 1887, the Surgeon General's Library was housed in the Army Medical Museum, which was located in the Ford's Theatre building where Abraham Lincoln was assassinated. Prior to the arrival of Billings in 1864, a printed catalogue of that library listed 1,365 volumes. Nine months after Billings was assigned to the library, a catalogue was printed listing 602 works that compose 2,253 volumes. By 1871, this list grew to 13,300 volumes. The accomplishments of Billings as the librarian of the Surgeon General's Library for thirty years represent the springboard, if not the genesis, of the National Library of Medicine, currently the largest medical library in the world, containing over eight million items.

The first catalogue of the Surgeon General's Library produced under Billings's direction appeared in 1873 and was followed three years later by the publication of *Speculum Fasiculus*, the precursor to the *Index Catalogue*. The first volume of the *Index Catalogue* was published as a quarto of 888 pages, covering the literature from "A" to "Berlinski" and presenting both subjects and authors in alphabetical order. The ultimate compilation of sixteen volumes by Billings and his cocoordinator, Dr. Robert Fletcher, provided the readership with the most complete bibliography of the medical literature up until that time and has continued to do so—albeit in altered format—up to the present time.

Certainly, the *Index Catalogue* had its forerunners. In the eighteenth century Dr. Albrecht von Haller, a Swiss anatomist and physiologist who is regarded to be the founder of scientific bibliography, collated bibliographies of anatomy, physiology, medicine, and surgery. Von Haller's work was supplanted by Carl Peter Callisen's "conspectus" of the medical literature of the last half of the eighteenth century and the first third of the nineteenth century. Both von Haller and Callisen, however, limited their bibliographies to books and pamphlets, whereas Billings and Fletcher included the additional and rapidly expanding category of periodicals. With the publication of the *Index*

Catalogue, scientists, practitioners, and students had for the first time access to essentially all that was available in the medical literature. The *Index Catalogue* expedited research and facilitated the acquisition of knowledge related to specific medical disorders and therapies.

According to Fielding Garrison, "under the firm guiding of Billings, the first sixteen volumes of the *Index Catalogue* were slowly evolved, year by year, forming, in the end, a definite world-record of the scientific endeavor of physicians in all ages and a permanent monument to his memory. No one has ever given to secular history or to physical science what Billings has given to medicine and the medical history."[7]

A year before the first volume of the *Index Catalogue* was published Billings and Fletcher initiated a bibliographic companion, *Index Medicus*, a monthly classified record of the world's medical literature, also arranged alphabetically according to subject and author. Currently, *Index Medicus* contains over sixteen million entries in its printed form and as an online electronic publication, and has been an invaluable tool that is accessed innumerable times each minute of every day throughout the world of medicine and science.

Billings retired from the army in 1892 and assumed the professorship of hygiene at the University of Pennsylvania and directorship of its laboratory of hygiene. He was in residence in Philadelphia for only one year when he moved on from the medical field and concentrated his bibliographic and administrative talents on a venue that is distinct from the realm of hospitals, hygiene, patients, and surgical science. In December 1895, Billings was appointed director of the New York Public Library, a position that he held until his death in 1913. The creation of the New York Public Library was expedited by amalgamating the bequests of John Jacob Astor, James Lenox, and Samuel J. Tilden. In his capacity as director, Billings was responsible for the planning of the landmark edifice that extends from Fortieth to Forty-second Street and from Fifth Avenue to the Avenue of the Americas (Sixth Avenue) in New York City. In addition, Billings supervised the recataloguing and physical distribution of the library's holdings. Eventually the multiple branches of the New York Free Circulating Library joined the New York Public Library, thereby creating the world's largest urban library system.

John Shaw Billings was one of the most, if not *the* most, honored American physicians of his time. He was elected to membership in many diverse societies and associations, including the American Surgical Association. His powerful and commanding physique housed the extraordinary intellect of a pioneer in the diverse fields of bibliography, hygiene, statistics, medical history, medical education, and hospital and library planning. The breadth of his contributions and accomplishments earns him recognition as a towering giant among American scholars.

—~—

The red brick hospital that Billings designed in Baltimore was the environment that William Stewart Halsted (fig. 22), unquestionably the most recognizable name in American surgery during the early twentieth century, flourished in as a surgical doyen. Halsted, however, presents an interesting problem for the historian in an atmosphere that is dominated by revisionists. While the major contributions of Billings maintain their significance, many of Halsted's innovations that were once regarded as irrefutable standards for years are now looked upon as anachronisms that have been transformed, replaced, or completely abandoned. The two operative procedures most associated with Halsted, the hernia repair that carries his name and the radical mastectomy that was once standard therapy for breast cancer, have both fallen into disrepute. Similarly, Halsted's revolutionary educational approach toward surgical residency that was based on a so-called pyramidal system, in which a limited number of chief residents rose to the top from a large pool of interns, is now also a relic of the past.

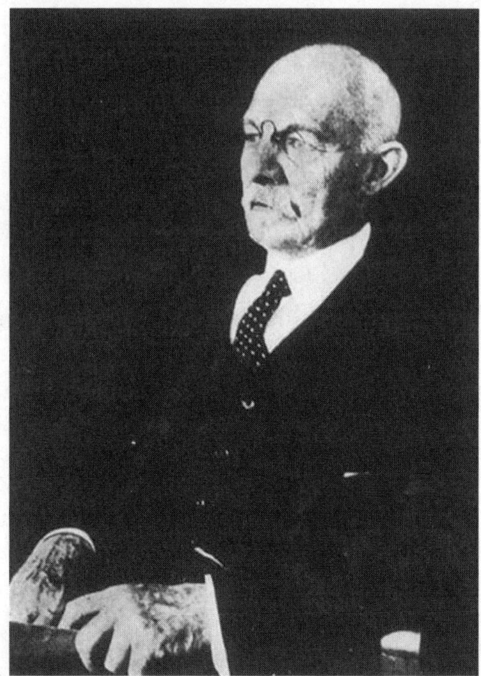

Figure 22: William Stewart Halsted. Courtesy of Alan Mason Chesney Archives, the Johns Hopkins Medical Institutions. Photograph by John H. Stocksdale, Baltimore, Maryland.

It would be, however, totally inappropriate in a compendium of America's most significant contributions to surgery to neglect the nation's dominant surgeon of his time and perhaps of all time. From the end of the nineteenth century and throughout the first quarter of the twentieth century, Halsted was the uncontested high priest of American surgery.

Halsted was born in New York City on September 23, 1852. He graduated without distinction from Yale in 1874 and immediately proceeded to his medical education at the College of Physicians and Surgeons, which was united with Columbia University in 1891. Halsted performed extremely well in medical school and was accepted as an intern at Bellevue Hospital before he had completed his medical degree. After graduation he served as house physician at the New York Hospital for one year, during which he devised a hospital chart system for recording temperature, pulse, and respiration with a series of dots that improved patient care. While at the New York Hospital, Halsted, prior to Reginald Fitz's classic paper of 1886, expressed an interest in performing an early operation for peritonitis due to "perityphlitis." He is thus credited with the first two appendectomies in New York City; both patients died, however, from complications of peritonitis.

Subsequent to those depressing experiences, Halsted embarked on a two-year tour of the notable surgical centers in Europe. In Vienna, he attended the surgical clinics of Theodor Billroth, the world's most notable surgeon. In Würzburg, he visited Ernst von Bergmann, who advanced cranial surgery and also established a protocol for aseptic surgery. In Leipzig, Halsted attended sessions with Karl Thiersch, who was noted for his improvement of skin grafting. Halsted then went on to Halle, where he met with Richard von Volkmann, who was the first to excise the rectum for cancer and describe the muscular contractures due to an impaired blood supply, which is identified by his name. Finally, Halsted was hosted in Kiel by Frederich von Esmarch, who developed a compressive bandage for establishing hemostasis, which carries his name.

Halsted's activities upon returning to New York City represent a period of development, between 1880 and 1886, in which his scientific inquiry, pedagogic capability, and technical prowess all emerged. He was appointed an associate at the Roosevelt Hospital, where he developed its first outpatient department. In the anatomy department of the College of Physicians, Halsted organized what was termed a "private quiz," an educational staple of the time. While the course work at the medical school itself was perfunctory and led to the acquisition of a doctor of medicine degree, the real education was provided by a group of faculty who were privately compensated by several students to serve as mentors who would coordinate a curriculum and dispense independent and private quizzes. Halsted's ability as a teacher was well respected and his private quiz group was the most highly regarded. William H. Welch, who at the time was a member of the faculty of Bellevue Medical College and later would play a most significant role in the life and career of Halsted, provided autopsy material and taught pathology for Halsted's quiz group.

In New York City, Halsted rapidly established his reputation as a surgeon noted for his indefatigability as well as his boldness and originality. In addition to his activities at the Roosevelt Hospital and the College of Physicians, he also worked at Bellevue Hospital, the Charity Hospital on Blackwell's Island, the Emigrant Hospital on Ward's Island, and the Chambers Street Hospital, the site where his first published contribution to surgery had its origin.

Halsted's surgical boldness is evident from two medical experiences within his own family. In 1881, when his sister in Albany was hemorrhaging after the delivery of her first child, he transfused his sister with blood that he drew from one of his own veins. In an era before the compatibility of blood type was appreciated, fortune smiled on Halsted when his sister rapidly improved and survived. A year later, he was again summoned to Albany where he operated on his mother, incising a distended gallbladder from which he extracted seven stones and drained a copious amount of pus. She survived for two years, thus constituting one of the earliest successful operations on the gallbladder to be performed in the United States.

The first paper to appear in Halsted's *Surgical Papers* (1924), which was a two-volume compilation of his published works, is titled "Refusion in the Treatment of Carbonic Oxide Poisoning." Presented at the New York Surgical Society in November 1883 and published in the *New York Medical Journal* the same year, the paper details Halsted's care of a patient at the Chambers Street Hospital. Halsted successfully resuscitated a man who was unconscious due to carbon monoxide poisoning by removing the patient's blood through tubing inserted into the radial artery, defibrinating the blood, exposing it to the air, and reinfusing it toward the heart (centripetally) via the same artery. The patient completely recovered in rapid fashion. The report includes two additional patients, one with hemorrhage and the other with septicemia (infection in the bloodstream), who Halsted successfully treated with centripetal intra-arterial infusions. In the first case he used saline and in the second case he used the patient's own defibrinated blood.[8] Consequently, Halsted must be credited as the originator of autoperfusion. His report antedates by thirty-one years the 1914 publication of Johann Thiess of Leipzig, who is usually considered to be the originator of that procedure.

It was also in New York City that Halsted fathered conduction anesthesia (anesthetizing by directly blocking nerve traffic). After the anesthetic properties of cocaine were described by Dr. Vasili Anrep in 1879 and applied in 1884 by Dr. Carl Koller to anesthetize the cornea and conjunctiva, Halsted began his own experiments with the drug. He demonstrated that if cocaine was injected into the central trunk of a sensory nerve, anesthesia resulted throughout the distribution of that nerve's peripheral branches. He also showed that the effect could be prolonged by impeding blood flow to the anesthetized area with a tourniquet and that the injection of saline into the nerve trunk, or as an infusion into a region, could also effect anesthesia.

During the course of these investigations Halsted and his coinvestigators experimented upon themselves by injecting and sniffing cocaine. Halsted's experiments led to a lifelong addiction that he concealed from most of his associates. Welch, however, knew of Halsted's problems and played a major role in Halsted's future care. The effects of Halsted's addiction first became apparent in 1885 and led to his initial hospitalization in a Providence detoxification center. After that hospitalization, Halsted never returned to his practice in New York City and instead elected to accept Welch's invitation to join him in Baltimore before Johns Hopkins Hospital opened. Over the ensuing years, Welch not only encouraged Halsted's work and regarded him as a protégé but also continued to assist with the management of his addiction, which eventually required a second secret hospitalization. There is a suggestion that Halsted's addiction to cocaine was lifelong and even extended to morphine.

Johns Hopkins Hospital provided an environment for Halsted's unrivaled productivity and his ascension to the pinnacle of the surgical field. His initial contribution preceded the opening of the hospital and came from his laboratory. During that time, Halsted was primarily concerned with the basic problems of wound healing and suturing of the intestine. In the realm of wound healing, he demonstrated the importance of avoiding an unfilled space when approximating tissue and the critical role of the wound's organizing blood clot in the healing process. His seminal demonstration regarding intestinal sutures consisted of defining the importance of inclusion of the submucosal layer (the smooth muscle under the intraluminal surface). During the same period, he studied thyroid operations in dogs and demonstrated that a compensatory growth of the remaining tissue follows partial resection. He also detailed methods of preserving the adjacent parathyroid glands during removal of the thyroid, thereby preventing the adverse hypocalcemia consequent to parathyroidectomy.

Johns Hopkins Hospital formally opened in May 1889 with William H. Welch as professor of pathology and de facto dean. In September of that year William Osler was appointed professor of medicine and physician-in-chief. A month later, Halsted was designated associate professor of surgery and Howard A. Kelly was recruited as associate professor of gynecology and obstetrics. Halsted was shortly thereafter designated surgeon-in-chief and on April 4, 1892, he was elevated to the title of professor of surgery. The dominant role that these four men played in the evolution of the hospital was recognized in the group portrait John Singer painted in 1905 titled *The Four Doctors*.

Transcending all aspects of operative surgery was Halsted's introduction of rubber gloves for use during operations, a contribution that includes a romantic element. The nurse in charge of Halsted's operating room, Caroline Hampton, whom he subsequently married, experienced dermatitis that was caused by her exposure to the mercuric oxide scrubbing solution. Halsted arranged for the production of thin rubber gloves by the Goodyear Rubber Company to protect her hands and arms. Dr. Joseph Bloodgood, one of Halsted's associates, was the first surgeon to operate invariably wearing rubber gloves, which was the beginning of a universal procedure.

One of the earliest appearing essays in the two volumes of Halsted's published works expresses his preference for fine silk sutures rather than catgut in order to reduce the tissue reaction and improve wound healing. This is in keeping with the universal theme of Halsted's credo that pertained to all operations, a theme that stressed a deliberate approach emphasizing safety. Many of Halsted's publications centered on the theme of intestinal anastomosis, emphasizing the role of the submucosal layer, the use of fine silk sutures, and a technique that minimizes trauma to the tissues. He was also a champion of applying the principles of asepsis and antisepsis (avoiding and treating infection during the intraoperative period) at a time that a significant number of American surgeons loudly criticized the concept introduced by Joseph Lister from universities in Glasgow, Edinburgh, and London.

Halsted's diverse interests reflected the nature of surgical practice before the age of specialization. His publications covered the spectrum of orthopaedics, plastic surgery, tuberculosis, and trauma. His dominant interests, however, concerned the endocrine organs, the intestinal tract, the biliary system, peripheral vascular operations, along with two issues that his name is most closely associated with—hernia repair and the radical removal of cancer of the breast.

In regard to the biliary system, both Halsted's personal and surgical lives were highlighted by episodes related to the biliary tract. Beginning with his early operation on his mother and ending with the two operations that were performed on him for inflammation of the gallbladder, and the subsequent recurrent infection of the bile ducts, he maintained a keen interest in that anatomic area. In remarks made during the discussion of a paper presented at the Johns Hopkins Medical Society in 1897, Halsted refers to three explorations of the common duct that he had performed with success on two occasions about four years previously.[9] As far as can be determined, these probably represent the first three such cases performed in the United States, an additional testimony to Halsted's courage and willingness to extend the limits of surgical practice. In 1898, he performed the first excision of a cancer of the ampulla of Vater (where the main ducts from the biliary system and pancreas enter into the small intestine within the duodenum), successfully transplanting the common bile duct into the duodenum. In 1919, Halsted underwent a removal of his gallbladder and drainage of his common bile duct. In August 1922, two of Halsted's disciples, George Heuer and Mont Reid, performed an operation on him for recurrent cholangitis (infection of the bile ducts) from which he did not recover. He died on September 7 due to intractable bleeding.

For sheer bulk of published material, Halsted's contributions in the field of vascular surgery exceed all others. In 1892, he was the first to ligate the left subclavian artery (main artery to the arm) in its first portion and to excise an aneurysm (dilation of a blood vessel) in that artery with success. He defined the cervical rib as a cause of the aneurysm. He also studied the effects of partial occlusion of large arteries in dogs and based on that work, he successfully managed an iliofemoral artery (the source of the main artery to the leg) aneurysm by partial occlusion of the iliac artery (the source of the iliofemoral artery), using a constricting metal band.

In the realm of hernia repair, Halsted achieved eponymic fame for the procedure that he first performed in 1889.[10] Although Eduardo Bassini of Padua carried out essentially the same operation at the same time, Halsted was not acquainted with it when he introduced his principles of repair. But, in a summary of his experiences prepared in 1922, Halsted graciously wrote: "I had not heard of Bassini's operation until his German article appeared—possibly about one year after my first operation; . . . Bassini unquestionably has the priority." In the same report, Halsted indicated: "It gratified me to note that in twenty years I probably had not had a recurrence"—a remarkable experience considering that prior to the modifications he and Bassini made, recurrence was a frequent event.[11] Currently, the "Halsted repair" of the inguinal hernia has been relegated to the past and has been replaced by prosthetic patches and plugs that obviate the need to approximate tissue and by laparoscopic repair.

Halsted's name is also synonymous with the so-called radical mastectomy in which the entire breast with the underlying pectoralis major and minor muscles and axillary lymph nodes are removed en masse.[12] In an era prior to the mammogram, when patients were presented to surgeons late in the course of their disease with large masses, Halsted's specific goal was a reduction in the incidence of local recurrence; he achieved that goal. To his credit, he continually emphasized the issue of prevention of local recurrence rather than cure.

In the twenty-first century, with an educated public attuned to self-examination and sophisticated periodic mammographic surveillance, breast cancer is generally diagnosed at earlier stages and local recurrence is no longer a frequent concern. Local excision of the breast tumor alone or perhaps removal of the breast in the case of larger lesions is almost universally performed, and chemotherapy and estrogen antagonists are used to treat what is now appreciated to be a potentially systemic disease. Halsted's radical mastectomy has therefore become a medical dinosaur. Thus, the two operations that Halsted is most noted for have been erased from today's index of surgical procedures. But, despite the marvels of advancing surgical science, Halsted remains the most innovative surgeon the United States has ever produced and unquestionably the most influential figure in the history of American surgery. Although his operations have disappeared, his surgical philosophy and system for training aspiring surgeons persist, albeit with modification, and have maintained America's preeminence in surgery throughout the world.

With the advent of anesthesia a half century before the inception of Halsted's career, it became possible to deemphasize speed and surgical bravado and instead champion the cause of safe surgery. Halsted's insistence on deliberate, meticulous technique that minimized blood loss and tissue trauma followed by precise approximation of wound edges to achieve optimal healing has been passed on to the ensuing generations of surgeons.

Halsted's initiation of a training program for surgeons is regarded by some as his greatest contribution. His goal was not only to train surgeons for practice but, more specifically, to develop teachers and mentors who would, in turn, train future generations of surgeons. In addition, he stressed investigation and continuous dialogue with the basic sciences. The desired end product of the training program at Johns Hopkins Hospital was that of a clinician-scientist of the highest standards. In this regard, Halsted was unquestionably successful. Seven of the seventeen residents trained by him became professors at the nation's most prestigious universities, spreading the gospel of surgical education.

CHAPTER 8:

PRODIGY AND PROGENITOR

[Man] is furnished with the senses, so as to be impressed with the property of things; by which means he gradually, of himself, acquires a degree of knowledge. But Man goes farther, he has the power of receiving information of things that never impressed his senses; and, if he has that power, it is natural to suppose that one Man has the power of communicating his knowledge of things to another, each giving and receiving reciprocally; which we find to be the case.

—John Hunter, "Introduction to Natural History,"
in *Essays and Observations* (1861)

The Halstedian system of surgical training that characterized the early days at Johns Hopkins Hospital successfully produced several leaders of academic surgery. The most notable was Harvey Williams Cushing (fig. 23), whose name became synonymous with the newly evolving field of neurosurgery. Harvey Cushing, born in Cleveland on April 8, 1869, was the son of a physician and the grandson of a general practitioner who emigrated from Massachusetts to the Western Reserve in Ohio during the first half of the nineteenth century. After completing a public school education in Cleveland, he spent four years at Yale (1887–1891), where he performed reasonably well academically but distinguished himself to a greater extent in athletics.

Despite Cushing's athletic potential, he was determined to continue the presence of the Cushing men in the medical profession. He ultimately decided to attend Harvard Medical School, perhaps because his older brother had preceded him at that institution. The younger Cushing's four years at Harvard Medical School were praiseworthy and highlighted by his first contribution to surgery—an "ether chart" to monitor anesthetized patients undergoing operative procedures. Cushing was motivated to develop this chart

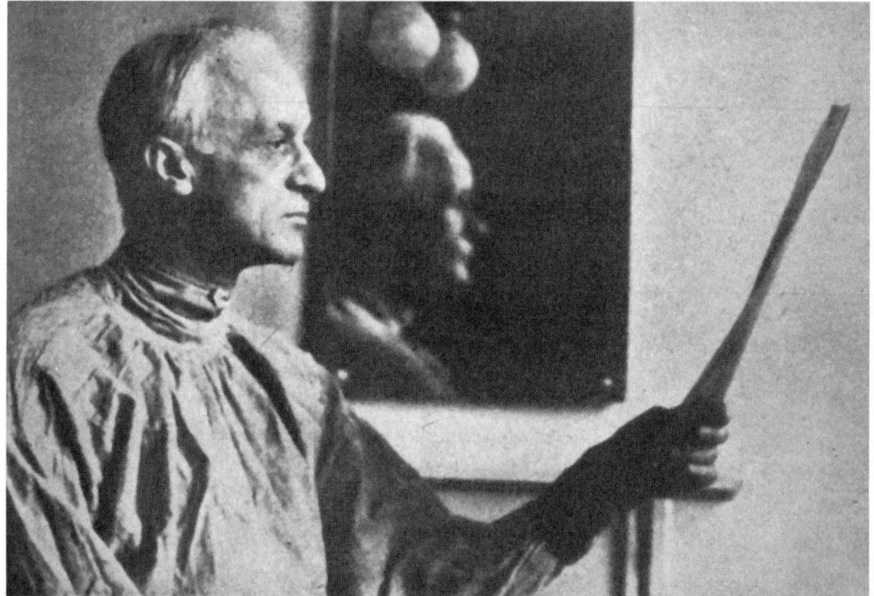

Figure 23: Harvey Williams Cushing. Courtesy of Yale University Cushing/Whitney Medical Library.

during his second year of medical school when a patient, to whom he was administering ether anesthesia by means of a sponge, inadvertently died. The patient's death, a result of Cushing's overuse of ether, greatly moved both Cushing and his classmates who witnessed the event. As a result, he and classmate Amory Codman introduced a chart that allowed continuous recording of the temperature, pulse, and respiratory rates during an operation in hope of limiting the occurrence of such deaths.

The earliest of Cushing's "ether charts," dated April 2, 1895, is preserved in the archives of Massachusetts General Hospital (fig. 24). Years later, after he had been exposed to the Riva-Rocci device for recording blood pressure in Pavia, Italy, Cushing brought an example back to the United States, allowing for a continuous measurement of blood pressure to be included on the "ether chart."

After graduating from medical school, Cushing served as an intern for a year at Massachusetts General Hospital. It was there that he participated in the early use of x-rays, less than a year after Wilhelm Konrad Roentgen announced his discovery in Würzberg, Germany. Cushing then moved to Johns Hopkins Hospital to train under Halsted. At Johns Hopkins he set up

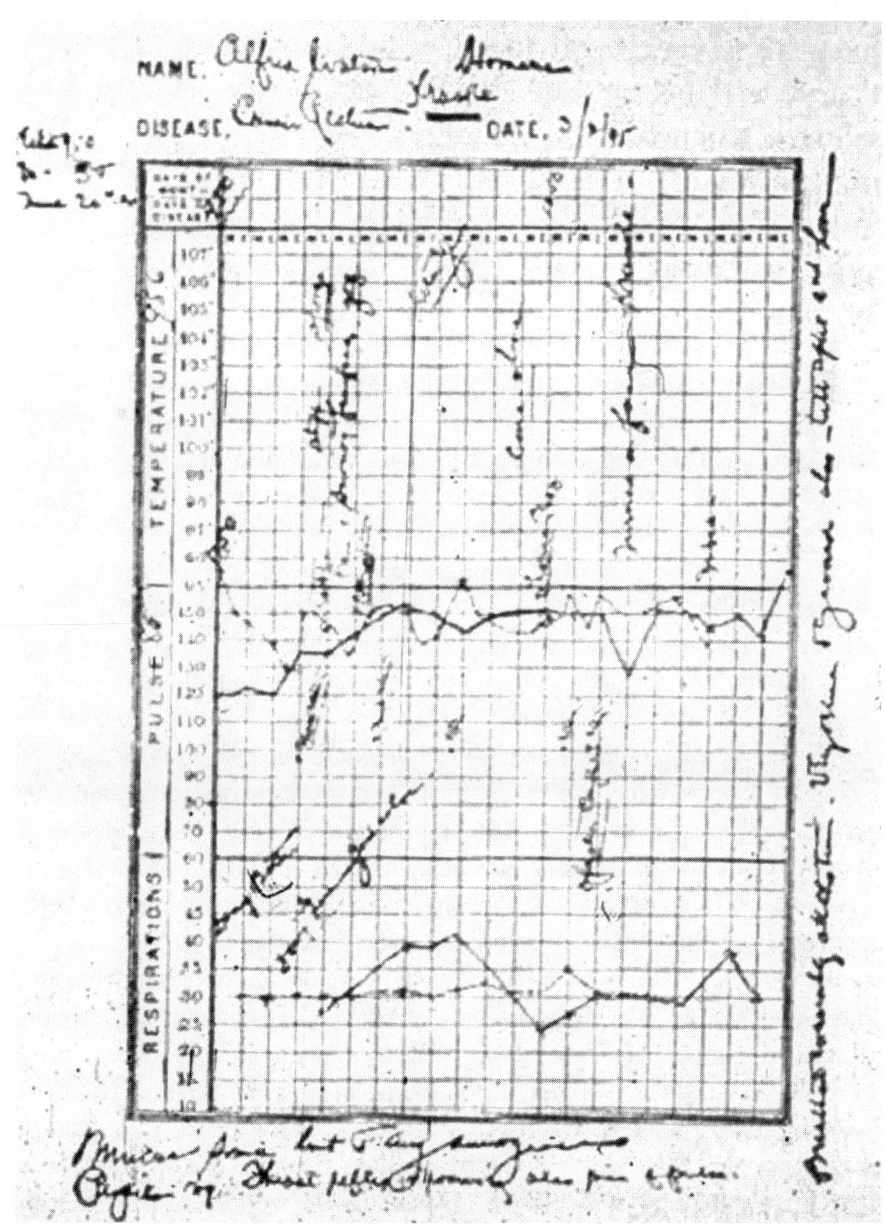

Figure 24: Earliest of Cushing's ether charts, dated April 2, 1895. Courtesy of Massachusetts General Hospital Archives and Special Collections.

an x-ray unit and reported two of the earliest cases in which x-rays were used for medical diagnosis.[1] One such case was a woman who had sustained a gunshot wound to the neck and developed paralysis on one side of her body, accompanied by sensory impairment on the opposite side. X-rays depicted the bullet in the sixth cervical vertebra. The report of this case represents Cushing's first publication in a scholarly journal.

Cushing's progress at Johns Hopkins was one of continual and rapid ascension. In the fall of 1896, he assumed the duties of an assistant resident in surgery. In 1898, he performed the first removal of a spleen in the United States for Banti's syndrome (anemia, splenic enlargement, gastrointestinal hemorrhages, and cirrhosis). The patient had multiple episodes of bleeding that were cured by the operation. In October 1898, he followed J. C. Bloodgood as resident surgeon and instructor in surgery. A year later, he was designated assistant professor of surgery and in 1902 he became associate professor of surgery, a title that he held until his departure in 1912.

During 1900 and 1901, Cushing spent fourteen months abroad. He specifically planned the itinerary so that he could study with Victor Horsley in London, Theodor Kocher in Bern, and Charles Scott Sherrington in Liverpool, because of their contributions to neurology (although, at the time, Cushing had no plan to specialize in neurosurgery). Horsley was one of the first to operate on pituitary tumors—which would become a major focus of Cushing's neurosurgical interests—as he standardized the procedures of laminectomy (excision of a vertebral posterior arch) and craniotomy (opening of the skull). Horsley also developed an operation to treat trigeminal neuralgia (intense pain along the course of the fifth cranial nerve), antedating another of Cushing's interests, and charted areas of the cerebral cortex. Horsley is thus considered by many to be the father of neurosurgery. Cushing, however, was disappointed by Horsley's technique and, consequently, abbreviated his visit.

By contrast, Cushing's stay at Bern with Theodor Kocher, who had published a classic treatise on lesions of the spinal cord associated with damage to the vertebral column, was most rewarding. Cushing was impressed by Kocher's meticulous, deliberate technique, characterized by an emphasis on maintaining the patient's complete homeostasis. At the suggestion of Kocher, Cushing worked in the Hallerian laboratory of Hugo Kronecker and conducted an experiment on a calf's head to determine if compression of the brain results in stasis or compression of the small veins and capillaries.

Cushing created a small window in the animal's skull in order to directly observe the effects of increasing intracranial pressure. He demonstrated that as the pressure within the skull increased, pressure within the arteries experienced a concomitant increase in order to remain above intracranial pressure. If intracranial pressure was allowed to exceed arterial pressure, the brain ceased to function and the animal died. During the same period, Cushing also demonstrated that frog muscle loses its responsiveness to neural stimuli when exposed to saline alone and required the addition of calcium chloride and potassium to maintain its functions.

He then proceeded to Turin, Italy, where he spent four weeks in the laboratory of Angelo Mosso, a physiologist who shared an interest in the consequences of increased intracranial pressure. While at Mosso's laboratory, Cushing developed the concept that there is a regulatory mechanism within the brain that responds to an increase in intracranial pressure and reduced blood flow to the brain, resulting in constriction of the peripheral blood vessels, thereby diverting needed blood to the brain.

Cushing completed his tour with a month in the Liverpool laboratory of C. S. Sherrington. During that time, Cushing participated in cortical localization experiments on chimpanzees, orangutans, and a gorilla to determine in which area of the brain various sensory and motor functions were energized. His surgical expertise was applied to perform craniotomies (cutting open of the skull) that allowed insertion of electrodes to measure electrical activity of the brain.

The interval between Cushing's return to Johns Hopkins Hospital and his eventual departure to assume a leadership role at the Peter Bent Brigham Hospital was one of extraordinary productivity. During that time, he crystallized his neurosurgical interests and established his presence on the national and international surgical scenes. In 1901, he attracted national attention for the first time with the Mütter lecture that he delivered in Philadelphia. In that lecture, he presented the work he had carried out in Bern on the relationship between intracranial and systemic arterial blood pressure. The lecture was liberally illustrated by his own well-executed, colored sketches. Throughout his career, Cushing used his artistic capabilities to reinforce his narratives.

At Johns Hopkins, in addition to his continued studies related to blood pressure, Cushing also focused on the effects of saline solutions administered to patients. In his 1901 paper, "Concerning the Poisonous Effect of Pure Sodium Chloride Solutions on the Nerve-Muscle Preparations," Cushing reported the results of the animal experiments in which he demonstrated that sodium chloride abolished muscle response to neural stimulation, but that if potassium chloride and calcium chloride were added to the solution, the muscle would reactivate.[2]

During his time at Johns Hopkins Hospital, Cushing was determined to develop his skills and reputation as a general surgeon with a focus on neurosurgery. He thus established the Hunterian Laboratory in which third-year medical students performed representative surgical procedures on anesthetized animals. In a 1908 publication titled "Instruction in Operative Medicine, with the Description of a Course in the Hunterian Laboratory of Experimental Medicine," the Hunterian laboratory was described.[3] Many academic surgical departments throughout the nation adopted this very popular educational experience. Skills labs that employed modules, mannequins, and mechanical devices, however, have ultimately replaced this approach, a change accelerated in part by the crusades of animal rights activists.

In 1903, despite his overt interest in neurosurgery, evidence of Cushing's desire to maintain a dialogue with all disciplines of surgery manifested in his formation of the Society of Clinical Surgery. This was a traveling club of surgical leaders who visited various clinics to witness operations and learn of the experimental and research activities of the host institutions. The Society of Clinical Surgery would provide needed diversification for many surgeons as the era of specialization began to unfold.

Neurosurgery, however, remained Cushing's primary passion. By concentrating his clinical activities in such a relatively new field, Cushing was embarking on uncharted waters. After all, it was not until 1884 that Francesco Durante of Rome reported the first successful removal of a brain tumor. Victor Horsley's first operation on the brain took place in 1886 at the National Hospital, Queen Square, London, only fourteen years before Cushing's visit. The earliest compendium on the subject. Antony Chipault's two-volume *Chirurgie opératoire du système nervaux* was not published until 1894. Thus, Cushing's opportunities for scientific advancement within the field of neurosurgery were limitless.

One of Cushing's initial neurosurgical interests was a new approach for the surgical relief of the severe, incapacitating facial pain known as trigeminal neuralgia, or "tic douloureux." At the invitation of W. W. Keen, professor of surgery at Jefferson Medical College, Cushing presented a paper that discussed the surgical management of trigeminal neuralgia by total removal of the Gasserian ganglion (the mass of nerves at the root of the fifth cranial nerve). The paper was published in the *Journal of the American Medical Association* in 1900 and is regarded as a classic both because of its textual and its illustrative detail.[4] This presentation led to Cushing's invitation to provide the section on neurosurgery, consisting of 276 pages and 154 illustrations, for Keen's highly regarded *System of Surgery*, published in 1908. Cushing's analysis of the areas of the face, innervated by the various branches of the trigeminal (fifth cranial) nerve, also remains a classic.[5] He extended his interest to sensory problems of the peripheral nerves, regeneration of peripheral nerves, and surgery of the spinal column.

During the early years of Cushing's experience as a brain surgeon, the number of operations that he performed was limited and the mortality rate was discouragingly high. By 1903, he had operated on a total of only seven cases. Coincidentally, in 1905, Amory Codman, the coauthor of Cushing's ether chart, reviewed twenty-eight cases of brain tumors operated on at Massachusetts General Hospital and ended with the pessimistic conclusion: "I may sum up the observations on brain tumor by saying that the reading of these records has made me personally feel that the chance of any success by radical operation was so small, that in any given case diagnosed as brain tumor, even if the symptoms gave evidence of more or less exact localization, it would be wiser to do an operation simply for the relief of intracranial pressure than to explore with the idea of removing the tumor."[6] In both 1906 and 1907, shortly after Codman's discouraging report, Cushing operated on only ten patients with brain tumors, with the results being hardly praiseworthy. By 1910, however, Cushing was able to report that in his last one hundred cases, there were thirty cures, thirteen operative deaths, and fifty-seven patients who had been palliated (alleviated of symptoms).[7]

From 1908 to 1912, Cushing focused on the pituitary gland, its physiology, pathology, and the surgical treatment of tumors that developed within the organ. He began experimenting on dogs and established that the gland had an important influence on a broad variety of metabolic processes. In 1909, Cushing performed his first operation for acromegaly (enlargement of the bones caused by abnormal activity of the pituitary gland) at a time when only one successful procedure had been previously reported, that one by Herman Schloffer of Innsbruck in 1907. Cushing followed Schloffer's approach and removed a portion of the anterior lobe of the pituitary. The patient enjoyed significant symptomatic improvement and lived for twenty years after the operation. In 1910, Cushing published a paper in the *Journal of the American Medical Association* introducing the terms "hypopituitarism" and "hyperpituitarism" that referred to decreased and increased activity of the pituitary gland.[8] By 1911, Cushing had managed forty-six patients with pituitary lesions, most of whom he operated on.

In 1912, his classic book, *The Pituitary Body and Its Disorders*, was published and evoked broad critical acclaim. In essence, the monograph is a detailed study of fifty cases. These cases emphasize that acromegaly is associated with excess hormone secretion by eosin-staining cells of the anterior lobe of the pituitary and is self-limiting, often resulting in reduced function of the pituitary gland. Cushing determined surgical intervention might be necessary to preserve vision that is threatened by impingement of the tumor on the optic nerve, or to limit the extent of the manifestations of the hyperpituitarism. There is also a detailed description in the monograph, accompanied by Cushing's elegantly executed illustrations, of the trans-sphenoidal approach (through the wedge-shaped bone at the base of the skull via the nasal passage) that he developed and made use of in order to expedite removal of the tumor.[9]

Harvey Cushing was offered the chair of surgery in several institutions including the University of Maryland, Jefferson Medical College, the University of Virginia, Yale University, New York University, and Washington University in St. Louis. After refusing all of the other offers, in May 1910, at the age of forty-one, Cushing accepted the appointments of Moseley Professor, the senior chair of surgery at Harvard, and surgeon-in-chief of the Peter Bent Brigham Hospital, which at the time was under construction and did not admit its first patient until January 27, 1913.

During the ensuing two decades, Cushing's academic career flourished. It included a vigorous surgical practice, many contributions to neurosurgical literature, the training of a significant number of surgical and neurosurgical leaders, and an expansion of his reputation. His progress in Boston was only interrupted by his activities as a medical officer in World War I, the subject on which his *From a Surgeon's Journal, 1915–1918* is based.[10]

Shortly after war was declared in Europe in August 1914, Cushing began to organize a voluntary unit from Harvard to go to France. In March 1915, Cushing and the Harvard unit left for the Ambulance Américaine, a five-hundred- to six-hundred-bed hospital in Paris. Following a short stay, he returned to Boston, only to once again leave for Europe in May 1917 to join the unit that was attached with the British Expeditionary Force at Base Hospital No. 5. He remained in France until February 1919.

While at Peter Bent Brigham Hospital, Cushing performed an average of four operations a week. In 1917, his monograph *Tumors of the Nervus Acusticus and the Syndrome of the Cerebellopontine Angle* was published.[11] With fellow neurosurgeon Percival Bailey, Cushing also published a monumental classification of brain tumors, based on 492 of their personal cases.[12]

Cushing had a continual interest in technical improvements that would facilitate neurosurgical operations and increase their safety. Early in his career, he championed the use of silver clips to control bleeding from blood vessels that were inaccessible to a ligature. In 1926, Cushing, in association with physicist W. T. Bovie, developed high-frequency electrosurgical techniques to either cut or coagulate cerebral tissue and thereby expedite the excision of tumors.[13]

In 1931, Cushing (fig. 25) performed his two thousandth operation on tumors of the brain. In 1932, a monograph was published that represented a compilation of his surgical life's work, titled *Intracranial Tumors: Notes upon a Series of Two Thousand Verified Cases with Surgical Mortality Percentages Pertaining Thereto*.[14] Improvement of mortality associated with the operation occurred over the years. Cushing's contributions to the field of neurosurgery continued to the very end of his tenure at the Peter Bent Brigham Hospital.

In 1932, Cushing described the syndrome that continues to bear his name, the manifestations of pituitary basophilism (excessive secretion of the hormones manufactured in the basophilic-staining cells of the pituitary). Cushing's work involving the clinical manifestations of central obesity, "moon" facies, dorsocervical (humpback) and supraclavicular fat pads, muscle wasting, thin skin, purple streaking of the skin, cataracts, osteoporosis, amenorrhea (cessation of menstrual flow), diabetes mellitus, and growth retardation resulting from hypercortisolism (excess of the adrenal hormone cortisol) will forever perpetuate his name in the annals of medicine.[15]

Cushing's contribution to electrosurgery, which had captured his interest from his internship days, increased the safety of removal of vascular meningioma (a lesion of the membranes covering the brain and spinal cord). His meningioma monograph, enhanced with his own operative sketches, was published in 1938.[16]

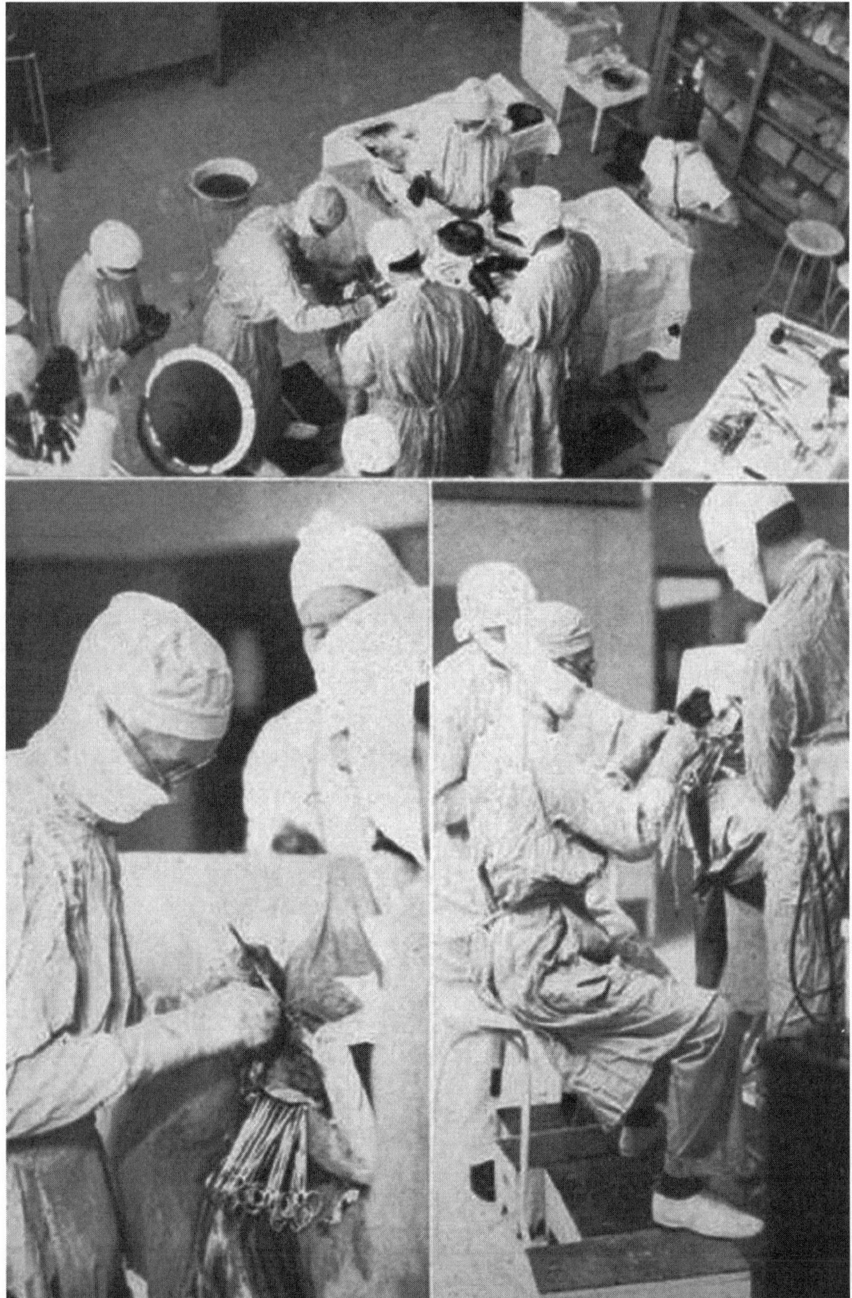

Figure 25: Commemorative photo of Harvey Cushing's two thousandth operation for brain tumors. Courtesy of Yale University Cushing/Whitney Medical Library.

In accordance with the rules that he helped write at the time of his appointment to Harvard, it was mandatory for him to retire at age sixty-three. Accordingly, he moved to Yale Medical School, where he carried the title of professor of neurology until he was sixty-eight. His seventieth birthday was celebrated in April 1938—he died six months later. His ashes were taken to Cleveland to rest beside his mother, his father, his brothers, and his son. Cushing's desk and library are located in the Sterling Library of Yale University.

Harvey Cushing is arguably the most honored American surgeon of all time. He was elected president of the American Surgical Association, the American College of Surgeons, the Society of Clinical Surgery, the Society of Neurological Surgeons, the Association for the Study of Internal Secretion, and the American Neurological Association. A list of the honors bestowed upon him by universities and societies throughout the world occupies four pages of print in John F. Fulton's definitive biography.

In addition to his extensive medical contributions, Cushing was highly regarded as a bibliophile and biographer. Cushing produced the definitive bio-bibliography (published posthumously) of Andreas Vesalius, the sixteenth-century Belgian physician whose original works Cushing collected over the years.[17] Cushing's other major literary accomplishment, for which he was awarded the Pulitzer Prize in 1926, was his biography of Sir William Osler, Johns Hopkins Hospital's first physician-in-chief.[18]

His literary identity as a bibliophile and biographer, coupled with his extraordinary medical contributions as a physician, surgeon, researcher, pioneer, innovator, mentor, educator, and administrator, create an image of the complete Harvey Cushing. Harvey Cushing is a prime example of the whole being greater than the sum of its parts.

CHAPTER 9:

VICTORY OVER VESSELS

I sent it through the rivers of your
blood
Even to the court, the heart, to th'
seat o' th' brain,
And, through the cranks and offices of
man,
The strongest nerves and small inferior
veins
From me receive the natural
competency
Whereby they live.

—William Shakespeare,
Coriolanus (1623)

The significant contributions of American surgeons that have been considered in previous chapters evolved during the nineteenth century and the early decades of the twentieth century. During that time, European surgeons and their well-established medical dynasties had dominated all aspects of gastrointestinal surgery. William Stewart Halsted and Harvey Cushing, however, represent a segue into the twentieth century during which American surgery advanced at an unprecedented rate toward supplanting European supremacy and obtaining its current position of world leadership. This ascension was due to the many diverse technical advances of momentous proportions made by surgeons within the United States, including refinements in anesthesia, application of the principles of antisepsis, antibiotic therapy, and an appreciation of the importance of maintaining or reestablishing homeostasis during and after increasingly complex operations. In each of these elements, American surgeons made significant contributions.

The twentieth century witnessed the dramatic birth and development of specialization in vascular surgery, cardiothoracic surgery, and organ transplantation. In each instance, surgeons working in the United States not only sowed the seeds for the birth of these specialties, but nurtured them throughout their growth. While these three specialties have achieved recognition as individual fields, there is a commonality within their technical and procedural elements that fosters a critical interdependence between them.

From a chronological perspective, each of these specialties evolved during the lives of today's older generation of surgeons, who proudly refer to the period that they practiced in as the Golden Age of Surgery. Significant advancements in the field of vascular surgery preceded the onset of cardiothoracic surgery, which, in turn, occurred before organ transplantation. Therefore, vascular surgery will be considered first.

The adjective "vascular" is derived from the Latin "vasculum," the diminutive for "vas," meaning vessel. Vascular surgery incorporates procedures performed on the peripheral vascular system, including all of the arterial conduits from the aorta as it exits the heart to the most distal small arteries within the body cavities, the extremities, and all of the venous channels that return blood to the heart.

The early history of vascular surgery within the United States consists of isolated case reports of ligations (tying-off) of major vessels proximal to aneurysms (dilations of arteries) due to trauma, syphilis, or the aging process. At this point in history, the aim of surgical intervention was to prevent life-threatening hemorrhage. Early in the history of the new nation, the boldness and reputation of the notable surgeons were mainly related to their accomplishments in vascular surgery because it was a time when, with the exception of Ephraim McDowell's removal of the ovaries, there were no abdominal or thoracic operations performed. Surgical anesthesia had not been introduced and the only targets for the scalpel or ligature were those that were relatively superficial and readily accessible.

The American surgeons' early operations on blood vessels stemmed from the accomplishments of London surgeon John Hunter. Although others had preceded him in the performance of proximal ligation of a large vessel to prevent massive bleeding from a diseased vessel, Hunter's classic ligation of the femoral artery (the main artery to the leg) in an anatomic location canal of the upper leg (which became known as Hunter's canal) was the major stimulus for early interest in operating on diseased blood vessels.

Later on, several of Hunter's pupils enforced the concept of proximal ligation. John Abernathy, Hunter's immediate successor, was the first to ligate the external iliac artery for aneurysm in 1796, an operation that he performed four times, twice successfully. In 1798, Abernathy also ligated the common carotid artery in the neck for hemorrhage. In 1805, Sir Astley Cooper, another pupil of John Hunter, ligated the carotid artery for aneurysm and also the aorta to prevent rupture of an iliac artery (the artery from which the main artery to the leg originates) aneurysm.

On the other side of the Atlantic, three of the most notable American surgeons in the early nineteenth century were John Syng Dorsey of Philadelphia, Wright Post of New York City, and Valentine Mott (Post's student), also of New York City. Dorsey, the nephew of Philip Syng Physick, was the first American to ligate the external iliac artery, in 1811, a feat repeated three years later by Post, who was professor of surgery at the Columbia College of Medicine (before it joined with the College of Physicians and Surgeons in New York City).

Valentine Mott received his MD from Columbia College in 1806 before going on to study with Sir Astley Cooper and John Abernathy in London and with John Bell in Edinburgh. Mott was elected professor of surgery at Columbia College in 1811 and became the first chair of surgery after the Columbia College and College of Physicians combined in 1813. He was the first to ligate the innominate artery (the right artery arising from the arch of the aorta and dividing into the right common carotid artery and the right subclavian artery) proximal to a subclavian aneurysm, in 1818. The patient lived for twenty-eight days only to die of exsanguination (blood loss). In 1827, Mott successfully ligated the common iliac artery for an aneurysm of the external iliac artery. In all, Mott is said to have performed one hundred thirty-eight ligations for aneurysms of major arteries, including the subclavian, eight times; the external carotid, fifty-one times; the common carotid, two times; the common iliac, one time; the external iliac, six times; the internal iliac, two times; the femoral, fifty-seven times; and the popliteal, ten times. Sir Astley Cooper indicated that Mott performed more operations on the major blood vessels than any surgeon up until that time.[1]

Well over a half century would elapse before the next innovation in vascular surgery occurred. That innovation took place in the United States at the hands of Rudolph Matas (1860–1957) (fig. 26) of New Orleans, whom many refer to as the Father of Modern Vascular Surgery. Matas was born on a Louisiana plantation and earned his MD at Tulane University before his twentieth birthday. During his long life, Matas was a professor of surgery at Tulane Medical School and served as president of the American College of

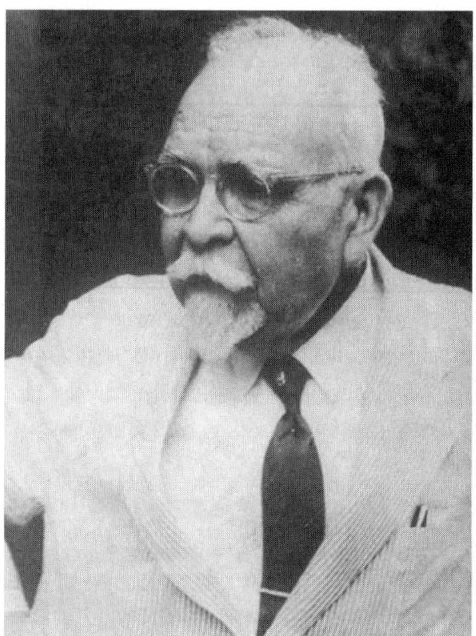

Figure 26: Rudolph Matas. Courtesy of Isidore Cohn, Jr.

Surgeons, the American Surgical Association, the American Association for Thoracic Surgery, and the International Society of Surgery. His revolutionary contribution to the field of vascular surgery took place at Charity Hospital in New Orleans on May 3, 1888. The operative procedure was actually a modification of an operation that had been described by the ancient Greek surgeon Antyllus circa 300 CE. Antyllus had ligated an artery above and below an aneurysm that was then opened, evacuated, and packed.

Matas was presented with a twenty-six-year-old plantation worker who had sustained a fine-shot wound of his left upper arm that had progressed to a pulsating aneurysm of the brachial artery. Matas initially followed the example of Hunter and ligated the artery proximal to the aneurysm, but this failed to permanently ablate the pulsations within the swelling. Therefore, he reexplored the arm and, when ligation of the brachial artery distal to the aneurysm failed to correct the situation, Matas opened the sac, sutured the openings of vessels that entered the back wall of the sac, and left the sac open. The patient recovered and returned to his normal life.

Matas reported his initial case in the *Philadelphia News* in 1888, but did not repeat the procedure for almost twelve years.[2] In February 1903, his classic article, "An Operation for the Radical Cure of Aneurysm Based on Arteriorraphy," appeared in a volume of the *Annals of Surgery.*[3] This report included four cases, the first being the patient who had been operated on in 1888. Two variants of aneurysmorraphy (repair of an arterial dilation) were also reported by Matas. In the first type, the sac was opened and sutures were placed from within to close the openings of the branches, in addition to closing the main artery, both proximally and distally. The other type provided for closing the openings of the branches from inside the vessel and obliterating the sac with sutures while preserving the main arterial opening and its flow. Matas assigned the term "endoaneurysmorraphy" to the latter procedure.

In 1940, Matas published his personal experience with treatment of aneurysms, including 620 operations and 101 endoaneurysmorraphies. The mortality rate was less than 5 percent and gangrene, a common concern, never resulted.[4] Adding to his impact on the field of vascular surgery, Matas performed the first successful ligation of the abdominal aorta, just below the origin of the renal arteries for an aortic aneurysm.

Beyond the field of vascular surgery, Matas also pioneered the intravenous administration of saline to treat a critical reduction in the volume of circulating blood. He was one of the first to perform laryngeal intubation for administration of inhalation anesthesia and was second only to August Bier of Kiel, Germany, to operate using cocaine in order to achieve spinal anesthesia.[5]

Almost a decade after Matas's initial operation on a traumatic aneurysm, John B. Murphy, the flamboyant Chicago surgeon who championed an aggressive approach to appendicitis, made his own significant contribution to vascular surgery—the first successful human arterial end-to-end anastomosis. In 1896, Murphy removed the common femoral artery containing a traumatic aneurysm and invaginated (ensheathed) the distal part of the vessel into the proximal end before applying sutures. He reported his experimental and clinical results in the *Medical Recorder* of 1897.[6]

Although Matas is referred to by some as the Father of Modern Vascular Surgery, his contribution was in reality derivative of Antyllus. It is instead more appropriate to equate the modernizing of vascular surgery with Alexis Carrel. In 1912, Carrel was the first Nobel Laureate for Physiology or Medicine to whom the prize was awarded for work performed mainly on American soil. It was his work on vascular anastomosis (suturing blood vessels together to maintain flow) and transplantation of vessels and organs that the award recognized. Previously, the only surgeon to receive the Nobel Prize for Physiology or Medicine was Theodor Kocher of Bern, Switzerland, in 1909.

Alexis Carrel (1873–1944) (fig. 27) was an enigmatic character who, as Charles A. Lindbergh indicated, "was one of the most extraordinary and controversial figures of his generation. Bearing a fame that spread around the planet, he was decorated and damned, often by the same people."[7] In many respects, Carrel was a scientific visionary, fifty years ahead of his time. He

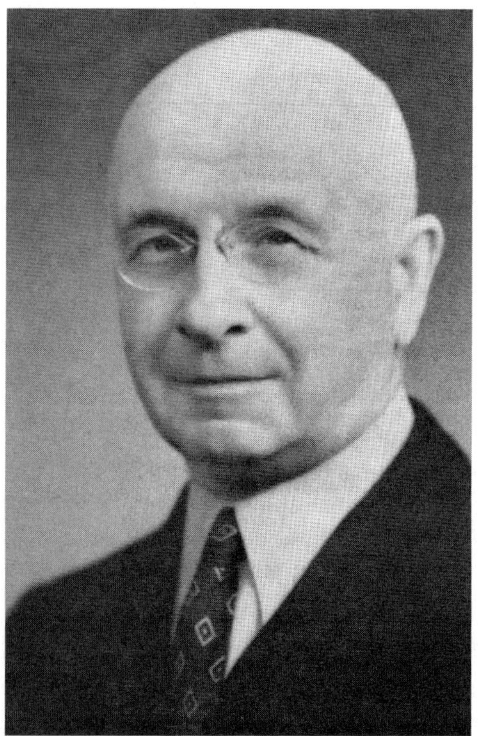

Figure 27: Alexis Carrel. Courtesy of Rockefeller Archives Center.

did, however, also espouse extrasensory perception and advance broad plans for remaking humankind. He also remained throughout his life a chauvinistic Frenchman, despite the fact that his research was conducted mainly in Chicago and New York City.

Born Auguste, he took Alexis, the given name of his father, when he was five years old, after his father died. Carrel received his MD from the University of Lyon in 1900, two years after he had served as a "prosecteur," teaching anatomy and experimental surgery. According to Carrel, his interest in vascular surgery specifically stemmed from the assassination of the president of the French Republic, Sadi Carnot, on June 24, 1894. In Lyon, Carnot sustained a knife wound of the portal vein (a large vein that connects the digestive track and liver) at the hands of Cesare Santo, an Italian anarchist. At the time, repair of blood vessels was considered impossible; this became Carrel's quest.

Between 1889 and 1900, several surgeons in Europe and the United States began addressing the problem of vascular anastomosis. Eugène Briau and Mathieu Jaboulay of Lyon successfully approximated the severed carotid artery of a donkey, using interrupted sutures placed in a fashion so as to evert the vessel wall and capture only the intima (inner layer) in the stitches. A year later, Julius Dörfler of Germany, using fine needles and a continuous silk suture that traversed all coats of the vessels, accomplished successful anastomosis between the severed ends of blood vessels.[8]

Carrel began his own work in Lyon and first reported his results in French in *Lyon Médicine* in 1902.[9] In that publication, he described his technique of triangulation for anastomosis of vessels (fig. 28) and indicated that, at the same time, he was also pursuing the transplantation of the thyroid, kidney, and pancreas using vascular anastomosis. This publication was followed by three more papers concerning his research conducted in Lyon before he received an appointment at the University of Chicago, where he conducted most of his work in association with Charles C. Guthrie, a physiologist at that university.

At the University of Chicago, the technique of vascular anastomosis, using the triangulation technique to minimize tissue trauma and consequent

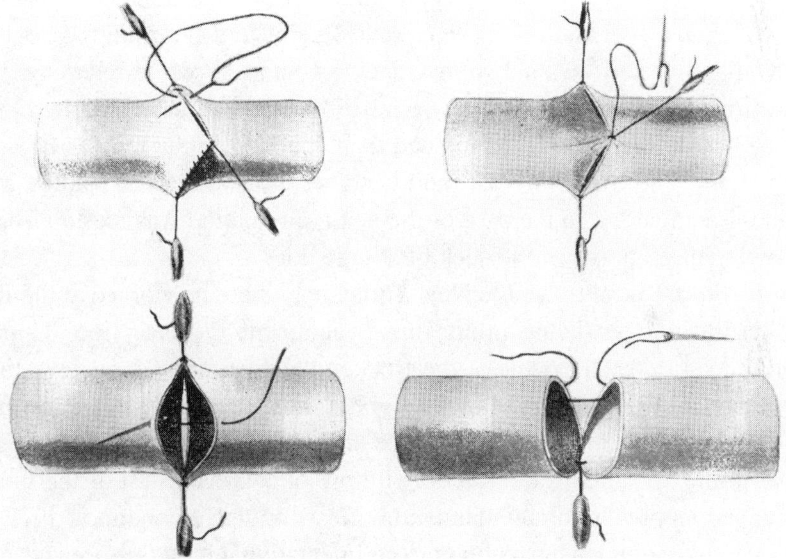

Figure 28. Carrel and Guthrie's technique for vascular anastomosis and insertion of a vein graft. "Les anastomosis vasculaired et leun techniqye operatione," *Union Médicale de Canada* 33 (1904): 52.

clotting at the suture line, was refined with the application of smaller needles and silk sutures. Transected arteries were sewn back together, arteries were anastomosed to veins, and fresh segments of veins were interposed between the ends of transected arteries to serve as effective conduits for the passage of blood. Within weeks of the venous transposition into the arterial system, the vein segments thickened to accommodate the increased pressure. Consequently, Carrel predicted that vein grafts would be used in the treatment of popliteal (behind the knee) aneurysms. That prediction would come true a half century later.

Carrel and Guthrie also autotransplanted (returning an organ to the organism from which it originated) the amputated hind limb of a dog by reestablishing the circulation that had been interrupted for over an hour. The first human limb reimplantation would take place at Massachusetts General Hospital in 1962, over a half century later. Carrel and Guthrie transplanted limbs from one animal to another with temporary surgical success but ultimate failure due to rejection. In 1902, in Lyon, Carrel had autotransplanted an animal's kidney from the abdomen to the neck. Renal function was maintained for a few days before the animal died of sepsis. This work was extended in Chicago by autotransplanting kidneys that remained attached to short segments of the aorta, vena cava (main vein returning blood to the heart), and ureter (channel from kidney to bladder), while retaining neural attachments in the abdomen. Normal production of urine resulted. Autotransplants of the kidney maintained their function for as long as two and a half years. The ovary, thyroid, and heart were also autotransplanted by the same investigators. In the case of the heart, circulation was reestablished by vascular anastomosis in the neck of a large dog.

In 1906, Carrel moved to New York City, where he worked at the Rockefeller Institute for the next thirty-three years, with the exception of a period during World War I. While at the Rockefeller Institute, Carrel investigated hypothermic preservation of arterial grafts. In the course of his experiments on the aorta, he defined the occurrence of limb paralysis due to lack of blood flow to the spinal cord associated with prolonged occlusion of the thoracic aorta and its prevention by maintaining flow through a conduit.

He also extended his realm of experimentation within the thoracic cavity, profiting from the development of endotracheal ventilation (administration of normally inhaled gases, oxygen, and anesthetic agents directly into the windpipe) by Samuel J. Meltzer and John Auer at the Rockefeller Institute. On animals that were anesthetized endotracheally, Carrel removed pulmonary lobes and intrathoracic esophageal segments. Carrel anticipated the field of cardiac surgery and described his concepts for correcting valvular and coronary artery disease.

Tissue culture also attracted the attention of Carrel's fertile mind, and his accomplishment in this realm gained extensive coverage in the popular press. He entered the field in order to develop methods of expediting wound healing. In 1910, Carrel reported that he had cultured organized adult tissue, including functioning cells of a chicken heart, an experiment that gained him the greatest notoriety. The viable cells that remained were actually generations of fibroblasts (connective tissue cells) rather than cardiac muscle cells. Carrel also demonstrated that cultured malignant cells maintained their malignancy.

At the beginning of World War I, Carrel, still a French citizen, was called upon by the French military to perform medical duty. His personal review of various French facilities led to his disparagement of the wound care that was being practiced in his native country. Through his association with the Rockefeller Institute, he was able to enlist the aid of chemist Henry D. Dakin, who was brought over from New York City to help establish a laboratory at Compiègne in France. Carrel and Dakin tested hundreds of antiseptic solutions in an attempt to find one that could act as a bactericidel, while excising the necrotic tissue without injuring the viable tissue. They finally settled on a solution of sodium hypochlorite—it would take the name of the chemist, Dakin's solution.

Carrel developed a method for administering the solution that allowed for intermittent irrigation of the depths of the wound. This method earned him the Legion of Honor from the French army and the Order of Leopold from King Albert of Belgium. In 1916, the Carrel-Dakin technique was accepted as the approved method of wound care by a surgical conference of the Allied forces. Dakin's solution continued to be used for wound care until the advent of antibiotics in 1939. An important by-product of Carrel's attempts to improve the management of infected wounds was his determination that the extent of contamination mandated microscopic analysis to quantify the bacterial count. After the war, Carrel returned to the Rockefeller Institute and continued with his diverse scientific studies that ranged from tissue culture experiments to an investigation of the effect of diet on malignancy.

The last of the significant scientific contributions that came from Carrel's laboratory involved a most improbable personality. In 1930, Charles A. Lindbergh (fig. 29), three years after his epochal transatlantic flight, began working with Carrel at the Rockefeller Institute. Lindbergh sought to develop an extracorporeal perfused heart that would sustain the patient while the surgeon repaired the native organ. Lindbergh was drawn to the project by the plight of a relative who might benefit from repair of her heart at a time when cardiac surgery was not a reality. Lindbergh and Carrel produced an organ-perfusion chamber, an apparatus that maintained pulsatile circulation of nutrient fluid

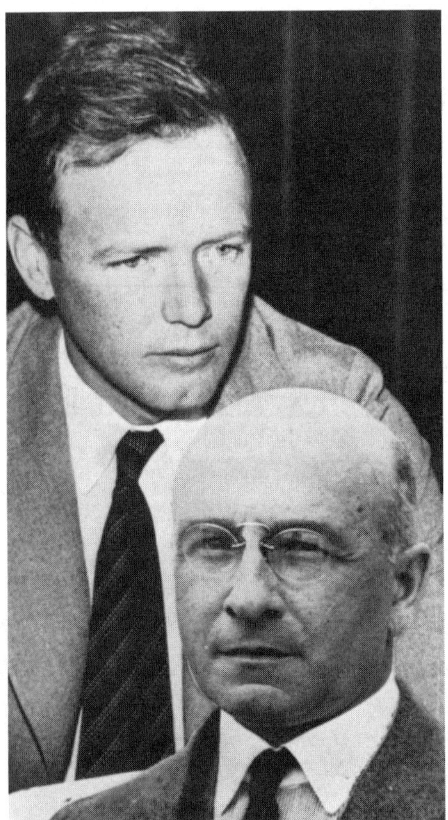

Figure 29: Alexis Carrel and Charles Lindbergh. Courtesy of Progrés de Lyon, Lyon, France.

under sterile conditions, while controlling the temperature and composition of the gaseous mixture for an extended period of time. The apparatus, however, was never applied to Lindbergh's relative. Decades would pass before the principle was applied to a patient with success.

Many of Carrel's investigations were performed on perfused (blood or physiologic fluid running through the organ) thyroid glands, measuring their secretion and stimulation. He successfully perfused the thyroid gland of a cat for eighteen days. Carrel's perfusion pump was a popular exhibit at the New York World's Fair in 1939. Hearts were kept beating for days. Perfused kidneys were short lived but produced urine for several hours. The perfused organs did well for varying periods of time, but eventually degenerated, leading to abandonment of the apparatus. This did, however, provide the principles that were incorporated twenty years later in the development of pump oxygenators for open-heart surgery.

In 1931, a unique honor was bestowed upon Carrel by the German ambassador to the United States. For the first time, the Nordhoff-Jung Cancer Research Prize was presented to an individual in the United States and, also for the first time, to a Frenchman. This award, however, perhaps came with a price, as Carrel, like Lindbergh, was criticized for his expressed approval of some of the tenets of Hitler's platform for Nazi Germany in the 1930s. Carrel left the Rockefeller Institute in 1939 and returned to France the following year. His last years were clouded by accusations of collaboration with the Nazis, and the French government conducted a search for evidence in order to prosecute him. While none was forthcoming, he was never officially exonerated before his death on November 5, 1944.

Carrel had perfected a technique for suturing blood vessels while minimizing the trauma and the consequent clotting within the vessel. The technique allowed for reestablishing the continuity of blood flow to the periphery. The next hurdle was to solve the problem of reestablishing vascular continuity if a segment of the vessel was removed or if the ends of a transected vessel could not be reapproximated. Carrel had shown that veins could be interposed into the arterial system but that exposure to the continuous increased pressure resulted in thickening of the vein wall and eventual closure of the conduit.

The next approach was to bridge a gap in a major artery, particularly the aorta, by a preserved homograft (isolated blood vessels that had been harvested from cadavers of recently deceased donors). The work took place in Boston and represented the combined efforts of Charles Hufnagel, at the time a surgical resident at the Peter Bent Brigham Hospital, and Robert E. Gross, who had previously distinguished himself by performing the first successful ligation of a patent ductus arteriosus (to be described in the next chapter), thereby marking the beginning of cardiac-related surgery in 1938.

In 1944, Hufnagel was trying to perfect a technique of dividing the aorta within the chest and sewing it back together. When he finally succeeded on a dog, he was confronted with a problem—when the dog's aorta was clamped for more that twenty minutes, the animal's hind limbs developed paralysis. He demonstrated, however, that if the animal was packed in ice to reduce its core body temperature, the complication was prevented. Hufnagel then began experimenting with the freezing of blood vessels. He removed the aortas from sacrificed animals and froze them in a mixture of carbon dioxide and alcohol in a tube, thereby creating a bank of vessels that were subsequently inserted into the aortas of other dogs. The work was first reported in 1947 in the *Bulletin of the American College of Surgeons.*[10] Hufnagel later contributed significantly to cardiac surgery and eventually chaired the department of surgery at Georgetown University from 1969 to 1979.

Hufnagel's findings related to vessel preservation intrigued Robert Gross, who had adopted Carrel's method of preserving the vessels for up to forty days in fluid tissue culture media at 4 degrees centigrade. In 1949, Gross and associates reported the insertion of preserved homografts from cadavers into the vessels of nine patients. Eight were to bridge the gap between the pulmonary artery and left subclavian artery in patients with tetralogy of Fallot (right ventricular outflow tract obstruction, hypertrophy of the right ventricle, a defect in the septum between the right and the left ventricles, and dextroposition of the aorta, i.e., located to the right of its normal position) and, in the ninth patient, to bridge the gap after removing a coarctation (congenital narrowing that impedes flow) of the thoracic aorta (see chapter 10).[11] Gross (fig. 30) succeeded William E. Ladd as professor of children's surgery at Harvard Medical School and became the president of the American Association of Thoracic Surgery and the first president of the American Pediatric Surgical Association.

Homografts also played a role in the revolutionary changes in the management of arterial injuries that were introduced by American surgeons. At the end of World War II, Michael E. DeBakey and Fiorindo A. Simeone published a treatise on the battle injuries of arteries in American troops during that conflict.[12] Among 2,471 cases of arterial wounds, there was an amputation rate of over 50 percent following ligation. By contrast, in eighty-one instances, suture repair was performed and in that group the amputation rate was only 35.8 percent. During the Korean War, with better triage related to the use of helicopters for evacuation, vascular repair became a more routine procedure.

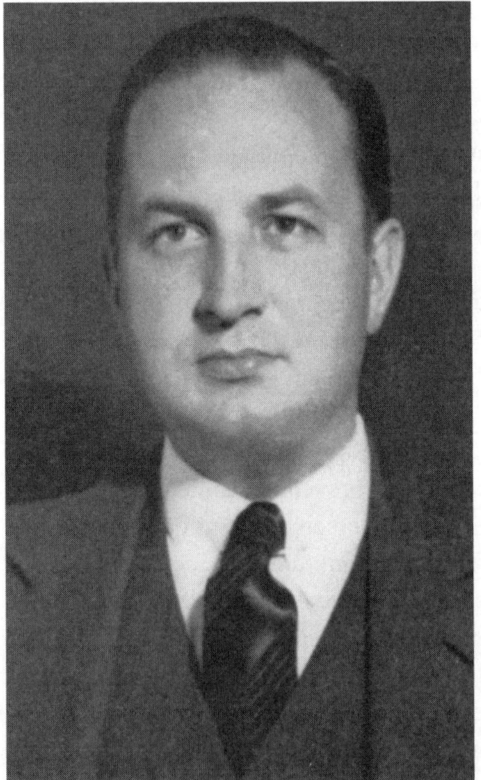

Figure 30: Robert E. Gross. Courtesy Edward G. Miner Library, University of Rochester School of Medicine and Dentistry, Rochester New York.

In 1953, Edward Jahnke and John Howard reported the initial favorable results for the repair of arterial wounds.[13] A year later, Carl Hughes published the results of 180 army cases with an 89 percent limb salvage rate.

Frank Spencer, serving with the United States Marines at the same time, reported similar results, often with the use of arterial homografts that had been taken from deceased casualties and stored in bottles of plasma in the blood bank.[14]

The homografts, in general, failed to afford acceptable long-term results and eventually formed aneurysmal dilations. Therefore, nonbiologic conduits to maintain blood flow through major arteries were sought after. In this quest, Arthur Voorhees, a Columbia University College of Physicians and Surgeons surgical resident, initially achieved the solution. In 1947, he noted a silk suture that was retrieved several months after it had inadvertently passed through a chamber of a dog's heart was coated with what appeared to be endothelium (the inner lining of a blood vessel). He speculated that a cloth tube might be used as a permanent arterial conduit by having its inner surface covered with native surface cells that would prevent clot formation and ultimate obstruction. He proceeded to develop a technique using a variety of cloths, but finally settled on vinyon-N, a material from which parachutes were manufactured. In 1952, Voorhees and his coworkers reported on fifteen animals in which prosthetic tubes had been placed into their arteries.[15] Two years later, the group published their successes in humans—one popliteal artery and seventeen abdominal aortic replacements.

Attention was rapidly directed toward improving the fabric. Hufnagel introduced Orlon, while others tried Teflon. The knitted Dacron introduced by DeBakey eventually received broad acceptance and, more recently, extruded tubes of Teflon (or Gore-Tex) have gained popularity.

The prosthetic grafts were first applied to the management of aneurysms. Charles Dubost of Paris is credited with the first publication, in 1952, regarding replacement of an abdominal aneurysm, in which he employed a homograft from a cadaver. Shortly thereafter, several American surgical groups reported many successes, initially using homografts and subsequently prosthetic conduits to replace the aneurysmal segment of the aorta. Prosthetic conduits facilitated the management of thoracoabodominal (involving the aorta within the chest and abdomen) and complicated aneurysms. In addition to replacing the diseased aorta, the major branch vessels—such as the celiac (supplying the stomach, liver, pancreas, and spleen), superior mesenteric (supplying most of the small and large intestine), and renal (supplying the kidneys) arteries—could be sewn into the wall of the tube to maintain blood flow to critical areas.

Whenever modern vascular surgery is considered, however, the name of one American surgeon comes to mind—Michael E. DeBakey (fig. 31). DeBakey has earned and enjoyed recognition for his contributions and leadership over the past half century. In 1932, he developed the roller pump for the heart-lung machine. In 1953, he performed the first successful carotid endarterectomy (removal of the inner layers of a blood vessel in which blood flow is compromised by atherosclerosis) and was one of the first to perform coronary artery bypass surgery. He introduced the Dacron graft for replacement of the aorta and sponsored the production of the artificial heart. As chairman of the Cora and Webb Madding Department of Surgery at the Baylor University College of Medicine, DeBakey operated on more than sixty thousand patients and was the author or coauthor of more than thirteen hundred peer-reviewed articles. He received the Lasker Award for Clinical Medical Research, the National Medal of Science, and the Presidential Medal of Freedom—the highest award a United States citizen can receive. At age ninety-seven, he suffered a dissection of the thoracic aorta, a condition for which he pioneered the treatment. On February 9, 2006, he became the oldest patient to undergo an endovascular repair for that condition. He recovered after a prolonged hospitalization and subsequently received the Congressional Gold Medal on April 23, 2008.

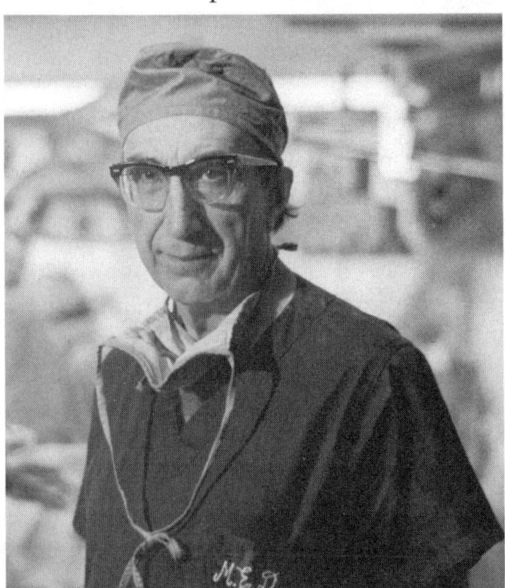

Figure 31: Michael E. DeBakey. Courtesy of Michael E. DeBakey.

In addition to treating aneurysmal dilations, vascular surgeons also directed their attention to occlusive disease of blood vessels that caused a reduction of arterial flow to critical organs and areas. The history of reconstitution of carotid arterial flow to the brain includes significant American contributions. Although the first successful operation for obstructive carotid arterial disease was performed by Carrea, Molins, and Murphy in Buenos Aires in 1951, it was not reported until 1955. They performed an anastomosis between the external carotid and the distal internal carotid arteries after partial removal of the stenosed area. In 1953, Kenneth Strully, Elliot Hurwitt, and Harry Blankenberg of Montefiore Hospital in New York City reported a patient with thrombosis of the internal carotid artery, verified angiographically (by injection of radio-opaque material into a blood vessel), in whom incomplete removal of the clot was performed. Because they were unable to achieve retrograde flow, they ligated and removed the involved part of the artery. The authors predicted the future when they concluded that a bypassing procedure, or thromboendarterectomy, should be successful if the occlusion is localized to the cervical portion of the internal carotid artery.[16]

The use of prosthetic grafts, particularly to replace the aorta, was occasionally associated with an infection at the site of the graft, often mandating removal of the graft. This required the development of a procedure that would maintain flow to the lower extremities in the absence of flow through the main aortic channel. In 1961, F. William Blaisdell, who chaired the department of surgery at the University of California, Davis, and his associate A. D. Hall published the solution. They attached a long prosthetic graft of Dacron so blood would enter it from the axillary artery to the arm. The graft coursed beneath the skin of the torso. The lower portion was bifurcated and attached to both femoral arteries, thereby maintaining blood flow to both legs.[17]

American surgeons also initially addressed occlusions of arteries supplying the viscera such as the kidneys and intestines. In 1954, Norman Freeman and associates first corrected renal hypertension by performing a thromboendarterectomy of the renal artery.[18] A year prior, Wiley Barker and Jack Cannon included thromboendarterectomy of the superior mesenteric artery (the main vessel to the intestines) in a patient undergoing endarterectomy of the aorta.[19] In 1957, Robert Shaw and Robert Rutledge reconstituted intestinal flow and obviated intestinal resection by removing an embolus (a clot that breaks off from one location within a blood vessel and travels downstream to another) from the superior mesenteric artery.[20]

The 1960s witnessed the appearance of two technical advances that had widespread applicability. In 1963, Thomas Fogarty, a research fellow in vascular surgery at the University of Cincinnati, published the description of a catheter that he developed for the extraction of arterial emboli and thrombi (attached blood clots within vessels).[21] The catheter is now used on a daily basis in many hospitals around the world. Dr. Fogarty was honored in 2000, by then a professor of surgery at Stanford University, as "the inventor of the year" with the distinguished Lemelson-MIT Award for several of his inventions (some unrelated to surgery).

In 1967, Dr. Julius H. Jacobson II introduced microsurgery for the anastomosis of small blood vessels.[22] The development of smaller sutures, miniaturized instruments, and a double binocular microscope with a five- to forty-power magnification and a sixteen-inch working distance led to success in bringing together the ends of the smallest blood vessels. Not only did this development expand the field of vascular surgery and neurological surgery, but it was also the genesis for the use of free flaps, or grafts of skin, and underlying muscle to cover surface defects, which formed the basis for finger and limb replantations.

Surgery on blood vessels is currently undergoing major technological advances with emphasis shifting to endovascular reconstruction of arterial flow. Endovascular surgery is a form of minimally invasive surgery that accesses critical blood vessels within the chest and abdomen from within peripheral vessels in the leg and arm. Large incisions and extensive dissections are replaced by almost imperceptible incisions and minimal disturbance to the patient. Typically, the artery in the groin provides access for the injection of radio-opaque agents that can be seen on x-ray or fluoroscopy and used to define the disease, along with providing a road map for its correction. The development of intravascular balloons for dilation and stents (tube inserted into a body's conduit to aid flow), which are inserted through a small catheter and guided into place where they expand to a predetermined size, offers a significant advantage over more traditional and invasive operations.

Once again, American contributions have led the way in this field. In this instance, however, it was a radiologist who merits recognition for primacy. After he had been appointed at age thirty-two as chairman of the department of radiology at the University of Oregon, Charles Dotter introduced interventional radiology. On January 16, 1964, he performed the first percutaneous transluminal angioplasty (passing through the overlying skin directly into a blood vessel to correct narrowing), dilating a stenosis of the superficial femoral artery. Eight years later, Charles Dotter introduced selective arterial embolization (inserting a catheter into a peripheral artery, directing the catheter under radiological guidance to the vessel that is bleeding, and injecting material to plug that vessel) for the control of gastrointestinal bleeding.

The birth of endovascular surgery is usually ascribed to the Argentinian Juan Parodi, who trained at the Cleveland Clinic to become a vascular surgeon. In 1990, Parodi, using a stent devised by Juan Palmaz, performed the first endovascular repair of an abdominal aortic aneurysm.[23] Over the last two decades, American surgeons, with the help of industrial collaborators, have made refinements that resulted in a now standard operative approach. The timing is appropriate because as the population continues to age, and there is a concomitant increase in the incidence of vascular disorders, more surgical procedures using techniques that compromise the older patients to a lesser extent are constantly being developed.

While disorders of the veins generally do not evoke the same sense of drama and immediacy as arterial disease, American surgeons have contributed significantly to an appreciation of problems related to the venous circulation and have introduced seminal operative interventions. Back in 1916, John Homans offered a classification of venous disorders and emphasized the importance of the veins emanating from deep within the leg and perforating through the fascia (membranous bands of connective tissue) to the subcutaneous area (beneath the skin). In 1938, Robert Linton described the anatomy of the so-called perforators and an operative approach for their interruption. In 1968, Robert Kistner introduced repair of the valve within the femoral vein to correct incompetency and the consequences of backflow.

In 1934, Homans defined the relationships between deep venous thrombosis (clot) in the lower extremity and pulmonary embolism (passage of detached clot from a vein to the arteries to the lungs)—a potentially fatal condition. Eventually, it became apparent that ligation of the superficial femoral vein (the main vein from the leg), introduced by Homans, was not the answer to the problem. Therefore, ligation of the inferior vena cava (the main vein returning blood from the lower part of the body to the heart) was introduced simultaneously by several American surgeons. In order to prevent the complication of stasis of the venous blood in the legs, which was associated with caval ligation, Frank Spencer initiated an operation on the inferior vena cava that allowed for the maintenance of flow while preventing the passage of larger, potentially fatal emboli.[24] This principle was applied with the use of a variety of external compressive devices that were replaced by internal filters. Currently, the most popular are variants of Lazar Greenfield's transvenous inferior vena caval trap that was developed in 1973.[25]

A complete consideration of vascular surgery includes the portal venous circulation that drains the gastrointestinal organs and becomes of surgical concern when bleeding from varices (dilated veins) in the esophagus or stomach develops. Once again, Americans played leadership roles in the modern era of surgical intervention for the management of that problem. Nineteen forty-five marked the beginning of the modern era with the publication of back-to-back reports from Columbia-Presbyterian Medical Center in New York City. The first report, by Allen O. Whipple, offered an in-depth consideration of the portal venous and splenic circulation and the collaterals, from which esophageal varices developed as a consequence of increased pressure within those veins. The aim of surgery was to shunt blood from the high-pressure portal venous circulation (over 250 mL saline) to the relatively low-pressure general venous circulation (less that 100 mL saline), thereby allowing the laws of hydrodynamics to come into play to correct the portal hypertension and cause the cessation of bleeding from tense esophageal veins.

He reported several cases in which a sutureless technique was performed to anastomose the portal circulation (by either an end-to-end attachment of the transected splenic vein or portal vein to the renal vein) with resultant control of hemorrhage from the esophagus.[26] The second report presented a technical modification using metal (vitallium) tubes to establish the connection between the high-pressure portal circulation and the low-pressure systemic circulation.

American surgeons have introduced several modifications of shunting procedures, but none of the decompressive operations is now frequently performed. Interventional radiologists have developed a technique for achieving the same reduction of portal hypertension without surgery. Under radiological guidance, a wire is passed from an arm vein and directed centrally into a vein that drains the liver mass and then into the liver itself, where it is then advanced into a vein that enters the liver from the portal (intestinal) venous circulation. A self-expanding stent is passed over the wire to establish flow from the high-pressure portal venous circulation to the low-pressure general venous circulation. This is referred to by the acronym TIPS (transcutaneous intrahepatic portal-systemic shunt).

As we approach the end of the first decade of the twenty-first century, we can anticipate a continuation and expansion of all aspects of vascular surgery, along with refinements in macroscopic and microscopic techniques that will be achieved with increasing speed.

CHAPTER 10:

BESTING THE CHEST

Surgery of the heart has probably reached limits set by nature to all surgery: no new method and no new discovery can overcome the natural difficulties that attend a wound of the heart.

—Theodor Billroth
Surgery of the Chest (1897)

Cardiothoracic surgery, like vascular surgery, is a specialty that evolved from the efforts of surgeons who had been trained to perform abdominal operations. The above quotation, which appeared in a textbook at the end of the nineteenth century, was written by Theodor Billroth, the world's most renowned surgeon of the time, and is evidence that cardiothoracic surgery was essentially nonexistent prior to its development and evolution during the twentieth century. Exponential growth occurred during the second half of the twentieth century, contributing to the designation of this period as the Golden Age of Surgery.

At the onset and throughout the development of cardiothoracic surgery, American surgeons were at the forefront. They have been credited with many "first" procedures and, more important, with the development of inventions and interventions that were essential prerequisites for the ultimate goal of correcting intracardiac defects under direct vision in a bloodless field. In order for the lungs and the heart to become the objects of surgical attention, it was first necessary to devise a system that provided for ventilation of the lungs and the delivery of oxygen to and the removal of carbon dioxide from the patient while the chest was open. The other obstacle associated with opening the chest is the loss of the negative pressure that is normally present within the chest cavity and maintains inflation of the lungs.

In 1899, Rudolph Matas first espoused inflating the lungs in a chest exposed to ambient pressure by combining a tube inserted into the trachea with a device to apply positive pressure.[1] Such a device was developed by

Joseph O'Dwyer, a New York City nose and throat surgeon, with a bellows system devised by George Edward Fell of Buffalo. However, it was F. W. Parham, Matas's colleague, who Matas graciously credited with the first application of the technique.[2]

Ernst Ferdinand Sauerbruch, initially working in the clinic of Johann von Mikulicz-Radecki in Breslau, Germany, and later in Zurich, Switzerland, considered positive pressure anesthesia, such as that championed by Rudolph Matas, to be injurious. Sauerbruch consequently developed an ingenious negative pressure chamber to maintain inflation of the lung in 1903. He successfully operated on patients with an open chest using this approach. The impact of the negative pressure chamber on thoracic surgery, however, was short lived—the end of its use was brought about by the work of Samuel J. Meltzer and John Auer at the Rockefeller Institute in New York. In 1909, Meltzer and Auer published their discovery that by creating an airtight fit for a tube inserted into the trachea, positive pressure ventilation could be effected and inflation of the lungs could be maintained while the chest was opened.[3] This advance led to the standard use of endotracheal ventilation for operations performed within the chest.

The first of the intrathoracic organs to be addressed surgically was the esophagus. Franz John A. Torek, who was born in Breslau, Germany, but was educated and practiced in New York City, performed the first successful removal of the thoracic portion of the esophagus for carcinoma. In 1913, Torek removed the thoracic esophagus, closed the lower end, and brought the open end of the cervical portion of the esophagus out through the skin of the neck. This was later connected by an external tube to an opening that was made into the stomach. The patient survived for eleven years taking pureed nourishment by mouth (fig. 32).[4]

Early in the twentieth century, surgery for diseases of the lungs concentrated on the treatment of tuberculosis. Surgical therapy usually consisted of draining the lung's abscesses or thoracoplastic procedures on the chest wall to collapse and thereby "rest" the underlying diseased lung. In 1922, Howard Lilienthal of Mount Sinai Hospital in New York was the first to report on the removal of one lobe of the lung, either as a one-stage procedure or as a two-stage procedure, with abrasion of the pleural surfaces as the first stage to adhere the diseased lung to the chest wall and removal of the diseased lobe as the second stage.[5]

In 1931, Rudolph Nissen, who would later gain eponymic fame for the

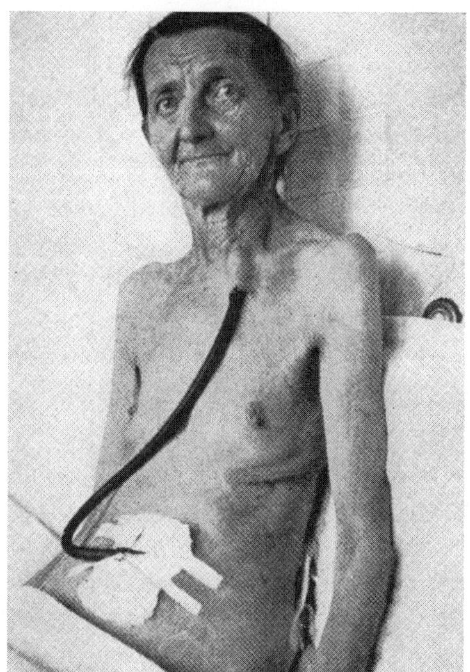

Figure 32: Esophagectomy patient from "The First Successful Case of Resection of the Thoracic Portion of the Oesophagus for Carcinoma," *Surgery, Gynecology & Obstetrics* 16 (1913): 614. Courtesy of American College of Surgeons.

operation he devised for the prevention of reflux of gastric contents into the esophagus, removed the necrotic lung of a twelve-year-old girl who had sustained a crushing injury to her chest. Taking place in Munich, this procedure, considered the first reported pneumonectomy, consisted of two stages. In the first stage, a tourniquet was applied to all the structures at the root of the lung, en masse, causing the necrotic lung to slough, while in the second stage, taking place fourteen days later, the lung was removed.[6] The patient was still doing well sixteen years after the operation. Eighteen months after the initial procedure, Cameron Haight of Ann Arbor, Michigan, used essentially the same technique with similar success.

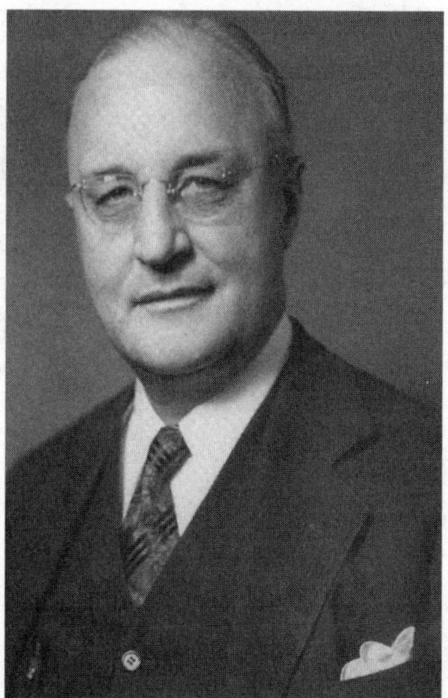

Figure 33: Evarts Graham. Courtesy of Becker Library, Washington University School of Medicine, St. Louis, Missouri.

Evarts A. Graham (fig. 33), one of the giants of American surgery, was the driving force behind the creation of the American Board of Surgery and served as president of the American College of Surgeons and the American Surgical Association. Early in his career, with Warren Cole, he developed a method for radiological visualization of the gallbladder. Most important, however, Graham is credited with the first successful pneumonectomy for cancer, using individual ligation of the hilar structures (the arteries, veins, and bronchi entering the lung).[7] In 1933, at Barnes Hospital in St. Louis, Graham performed the operation on James Gilmore, an obstetrician who lived thirty-four years after the surgery, outliving the surgeon, who, ironically, died of lung cancer after devoting his later years to eradicating the use of tobacco.

Alfred Blalock (fig. 34), the chair of surgery at Johns Hopkins Hospital from 1941 to 1964, is universally recognized for his contribution to cardiac surgery. Another of his significant contributions to thoracic surgery, however, rarely receives attention. He was the first to demonstrate an association between the neuromuscular disorder myasthenia gravis and the thymus gland, located immediately posterior to the sternum. This occurred when Blalock removed the thymus from a patient who coincidentally had the classic muscular weakness of myasthenia gravis. Blalock noted marked improvement of the patient's symptoms postoperatively. Although the initial patient with the thymic tumor and myasthenia gravis was operated on in 1936, the surgical concept was introduced in Blalock's 1941 publication that

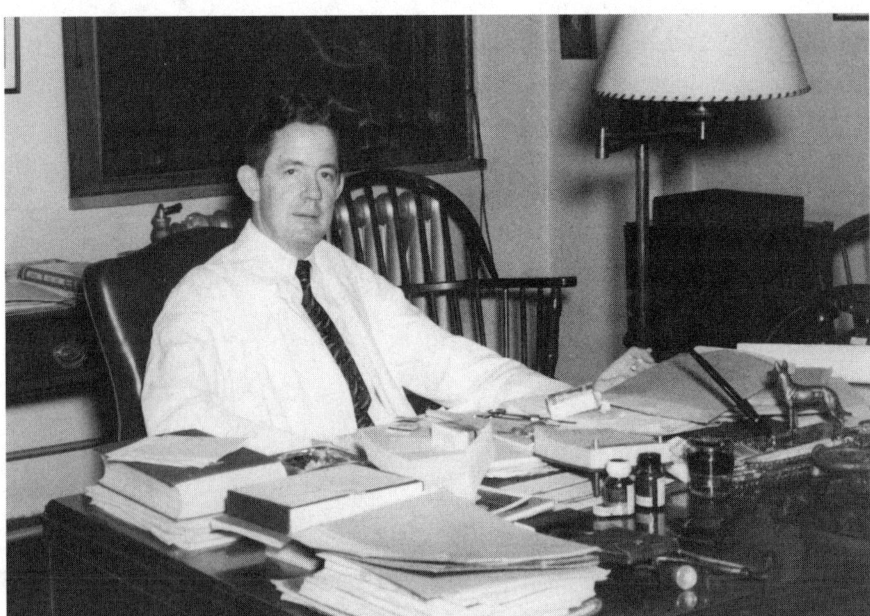

Figure 34: Alfred Blalock. Courtesy of the Alan Mason Chesney Archives, Johns Hopkins Medical Institutions, Baltimore, Maryland.

described a series of cases in which removal of the gland effected improvement of the symptoms—this eventually led to the procedure's widespread application.[8]

For both emotional and practical reasons, operations on the heart represented a Holy Grail of sorts for surgeons throughout the world. During the early history of surgery, the heart was considered an organ for which the Latin phrase "noli me tangere" (don't touch me) applied. As far as cardiac surgery is concerned, in no other field, with the exception of organ transplantation, was the American influence so dominant.

In 1868, Georg Fischer of Hanover, Germany, published a comprehensive review of cardiac wounds that generally had been treated expectantly, but with only 10 percent surviving. In the last decade of the nineteenth century, two American surgeons became the first to successfully suture knife wounds of the pericardium (the lining of the sac surrounding the heart itself), but neither operation necessitated placing sutures in the heart itself.

On September 6, 1891, in St. Louis, H. C. Dalton sutured a pericardial stab wound, but he did not report his success until 1895.[9] Dalton was operating in the chest of a young man in order to control bleeding from an artery severed by a fractured rib when he encountered a laceration of the pericardium. As Dalton stated in his article: "I had no precedent to guide me, no authority to uphold me in attempting to sew up this wound over a heart that was beating at the rate of 140 per minute."

Without knowledge of Dalton's experience, Daniel Hale Williams, an African American surgeon working at Provident Hospital in Chicago, performed a similar procedure in 1893. Williams's patient sustained an inch-long knife wound of the chest to the left of the sternum. As the patient progressively deteriorated, Williams proceeded to operate without known precedence. The surgeon's written report stated:

> A small punctured wound of the heart about one-tenth of an inch in length and about one-half of an inch to the right of the right coronary artery between two of its lateral branches was seen. The wound in the pericardium was about one and a half inches in length. There was no hemorrhage from the heart or pericardium. The edges of the pericardium were held by long smooth forceps and a continuous suture of fine catgut was made.[10]

The patient survived for fifty years after the operation, outliving the surgeon.

In September 1896, Ludwig Rehn of Frankfurt, Germany, closed a one-and-a-half-inch wound of the right ventricle with three sutures, thus becoming the first to operate with success directly on the heart. The first successful cardiac operation in the United States occurred on September 14, 1902, when Luther L. Hill in Montgomery, Alabama, drained a large accumulation of blood from the pericardial cavity and closed a three-eighths-of-an-inch bleeding laceration of the heart with a single catgut suture.[11] The patient was a thirteen-year-old boy and the operation was performed on a kitchen table using kerosene lighting. Dr. Luther L. Hill's own son, Lister, became well known as a senator from Alabama with an interest in the betterment of healthcare within the nation.

The history of cardiac surgery is appropriately defined by two distinct periods, divided by the introduction of reliable pump-oxygenation or extracorporeal circulation. The pre–pump oxygenation period was characterized by sporadic surgical incursions, generally accompanied by frustration and unacceptable mortality rates. The surgical efforts were heroic at times and, at other times, represented surgical hubris. The operations devised were initially directed at accomplishing repair of acquired and congenital lesions within the heart, but without direct visualization, which at that time was unattainable. In retrospect, many of the operations were ingenious, but few were consistently effective and most are now regarded as relics of the past. Cardiac surgery during the pre-pump period also concentrated on lesions outside the heart that directly affected cardiac function. Throughout that era, the contributions of American surgeons were significant.

A chronological review of the pre–pump oxygenation period generally begins with isolated attempts at improving the status of diseased heart valves, frequently a consequence of rheumatic heart disease. In the first quarter of the twentieth century, the reported procedures had little impact. The attempt in Paris by Eugène Doyen at sectioning the orifice of the pulmonary valve in 1913, and Théodore Tuffier's dilation of the aortic valve through the aortic wall a year later, could not be replicated. In 1923, at Peter Bent Brigham Hospital in Boston, Elliot Cutler became the first to operate on the mitral valve (a bicuspid structure so-named because it resembles a bishop's miter) located between the left atrium and the left ventricle. He inserted a cutting instrument, termed a valvulotome, into the apex of the left ventricle of a young girl and attempted to divide the cusps of a scarred and thickened mitral valve with an instrument known as a tenotome.[12] The patient improved to some extent but died in four and a half years. Cutler and his associate Claude Beck subsequently operated on six more patients using a similar procedure, at times with a modified instrument. None of the patients survived.

At the same time, Duff Allen and Evarts Graham at Washington University in St. Louis devised a cardioscope to provide direct visualization of the mitral valve and inserted the instrument into the left auricle of a young woman who immediately died, putting an end to that approach. Sir Henry Souttar's successful finger fracture of the mitral valve was first performed in 1925 at London Hospital. Despite the fact that the patient lived for seven years, a mitral valve procedure was not performed again for over two decades. Henry Souttar wrote in a letter to his Boston colleague Dwight Harken: "I did not repeat the operation because I could not get another case. Although my patient made an uninterrupted recovery the Physicians declared that it was all nonsense and in fact that the operation was unjustifiable. In fact it is of no use to be ahead of one's time."[13]

Before the mitral valve was revisited surgically, two operations on congenital cardiac lesions opened a new era. Progress in elective cardiac surgery proceeded in a centripetal direction, coursing from outside the heart to the interior. The first focus was on a small channel (2 to 8 mm long with a diameter of 4 to 12 mm), the ductus arteriosus, which provides flow from the main pulmonary artery to the upper descending thoracic aorta during the fetal period and normally closes spontaneously at birth. If the channel remains open, there is the potential that congestive heart failure or bacterial infection within the ductus or the heart will develop.

The story of the ligation of a patent ductus arteriosus actually began in 1907 when John Munro, chief of surgery at Boston City Hospital, was the first to publish a proposal to correct the defect.[14] In 1937, John W. Strieder, at Massachusetts Memorial Hospital in Boston, was the first to attempt to close a patent ductus arteriosus. The patient was a young woman with bacterial endocarditis. Complete closure was not achieved and the patient died five days after the operation. In the same city, seventeen months later at Boston Children's Hospital, Robert Edward Gross successfully closed the ductus arteriosus of a seven-year-old girl by ligating the structure with a single silk suture.[15]

Gross had worked out the principles and technical aspects of the procedure in the laboratory and the timing of the procedure, it is purported, was not a coincidence. The daring operation took place in August while the chief of surgery at Boston Children's Hospital, Dr. William E. Ladd, was away on vacation. The story is told that shortly after the success, Ladd met Gross and asked how things were at the hospital during his vacation. Gross stated that nothing unusual had happened. When Ladd found out what did happen regarding the operation, he was furious with Gross for performing the procedure without his permission. The operation was reported in 1939, and the procedure was later modified by dividing the ductus and closing the two ends.

Gross also had an early interest in the excision of coarctation (congenital narrowing) of the thoracic aorta with reapproximation of the cut ends in order to prevent or correct the consequent elevated blood pressure proximal to lesion. Although priority must be granted to Clarence Crafoord and Gustav Nylin of Sweden for initial success in October 1944, Gross had begun experimenting on correction of the disorder earlier,[16] and he finally achieved clinical success in June 1945, independent of the Swedish group.[17] Gross maintained that Crafoord had learned the technique in his laboratory.[18] In 1948, Gross was the first to use a cadaver's aortic homograft replacement successfully to bridge the gap of a removed coarctation in a seven-year-old boy.[19]

The successful ligation of the ductus arteriosus and removal of coarctation of the aorta were certainly significant, but they did not evoke the widespread excitement that attended the report of the successful operation that came to be known as the Blalock-Taussig procedure (subclavian artery–pulmonary artery anastomosis). This reaction was understandable because the Blalock-Taussig procedure was more complex and the conversion of markedly debilitated "blue babies" to more vigorous children was both readily apparent and very dramatic.

The "blue babies" with tetralogy of Fallot, a congenital heart defect, are pathetic images. On November 29, 1944, at Johns Hopkins Hospital Alfred Blalock successfully performed the operation that bears his name for the first time.[20] The first patient was a fifteen-month-old girl who weighed only ten pounds. Helen Taussig, the pediatrician who cared for the patient, indicated that the lack of pulmonary blood flow was a critical element. Vivien Thomas, an African American laboratory technician who helped pioneer the procedure in the laboratory, stood by Dr. Blalock during the procedure. The chief resident, William P. Longmire Jr., assisted, while Denton A. Cooley, a junior resident at the time, administered intravenous fluids. Dr. Longmire would later create and develop the department of surgery at the University of California, Los Angeles, and become a national leader in surgery. Dr. Cooley became a world-renowned and inventive cardiac surgeon. Vivien Thomas received an honorary doctor of laws from Johns Hopkins University.

The operation, which consisted of shunting the flow from the subclavian artery to the pulmonary artery, provided marked improvement for the patient, who died six months later after a second procedure. Long-term success was achieved in February 1945 with two patients—the first operation replicated the previous one, while, in the second instance, the procedure was changed. An end-to-side anastomosis was performed between the innominate artery and the right pulmonary artery. In May 1945, Blalock and Taussig's classic paper appeared in print. Subsequently, Blalock, bearing the mantle of a conquering hero, toured Great Britain and Europe and was integral to the spread of cardiac surgery to those lands.

Blalock was the best-known surgeon of the first half of the twentieth century in part due to the cadre of surgical leaders whom he trained, including the revered names of Mark M. Ravitch, Kenneth L. Pickrell, Herbert E. Sloan Jr., William P. Longmire Jr., H. William Scott Jr., C. Rollins Hanlon, William H. Muller Jr., Denton A. Cooley, Henry T. Bahnson, Andrew Glenn Morrow, David C. Sabiston Jr., Jerome Harold Kay, James V. Maloney Jr., Frank C. Spencer, G. Rainey Williams Jr., J. Alex Haller Jr., James R. Jude, Charles R. Hatcher Jr., Clarence S. Weldon, Lazar Greenfield, and Paul Ebert. All went on to become chairs of surgery or surgical divisions. In regard to the genesis of surgeons, Alfred Blalock can be compared to the "big bang" that created the universe of stars.

It was also at Johns Hopkins that much of the basic research was carried out on the electrical activity responsible for stimulating the muscles of the heart to contract and relax. Specific investigation of ventricular fibrillation was conducted in the 1930s and 1940s by the engineer William Kouwenhoven. Claude Beck was the first surgeon to become interested in the problem in the mid-1930s. In 1947, after several failures, Beck performed the first successful electrical defibrillation on a human in Cleveland.[21] Throughout the ensuing years, American contributions would continue to lead the world in the management of electrical activity disorders of the heart.

In 1952, Paul Zoll, working at Beth Israel Hospital in Boston, based on the contributions of John Callaghan and Wilfred Bigelow of Toronto, was the first to apply external stimulation to the heart in order to reverse ventricular fibrillation and cardiac standstill.[22] He was assisted by Howard Frank, the surgeon who subsequently performed the first direct placement of an electrode into the heart muscle and the implantation of the first miniaturized generator. Zoll went on to develop a noninvasive pacing system and the first clinically applicable cardiac monitors to follow the course of electrical activity over extended periods of time.

In 1957, at the University of Minnesota, C. Walton Lillehei and Vincent Gott performed cardiac pacing successfully through a myocardial wire placed during an operation on a three-year-old girl, who developed heart block during the repair of a tetralogy of Fallot. Subsequently, if temporary heart block occurred during the operation, Lillehei would routinely leave a wire in the myocardium of the right ventricle so that the patient could be paced temporarily through the closed chest.[23]

The first totally implanted pacemaker was inserted by Åke Senning of Sweden in 1959. A year later, William Chardack of Buffalo inserted the first fully implantable, unobtrusive, fixed-rate pacing system that had been developed by the engineer Wilson Greatbatch.[24] In 1961, Adrian Kantrowitz, at Maimonides Hospital in Brooklyn, reported his experience with a totally implantable pacemaker, the rate of which was controlled through the skin by an external transmitter.[25]

In 1980, continuing in the realm of electrophysiology of the heart, M. Mirowski and associates reported the first three patients in whom potentially lethal ventricular arrhythmias were terminated by the thoracic implantation of an automatic defibrillator with a pulse generator positioned in a subcutaneous pocket.[26]

Surgery for the ablation of arrhythmias began at Duke University in 1968, when Will Sealy successfully divided a right atrial free-wall accessory intrinsic electrical pathway in a patient with the paroxysmal tachycardia (burst of rapid heartbeats) of the Wolff-Parkinson-White syndrome.[27] James L. Cox, a pupil of Will Sealy, went on to devise the Maze procedure, a complex operation in which the electrical pathways within the heart were divided for the treatment of medically refractory atrial flutter and fibrillation.[28]

In returning to a chronological consideration—after Alfred Blalock dramatically rekindled interest in cardiac surgery in 1945—attention was then directed toward the surgical correction of heart valve disorders that were a common consequence of rheumatic heart disease and atherosclerosis. As indicated previously, this represented a hiatus of more than twenty years after the initial temporary success that had been achieved by Souttar in 1925. Because of the absence of the ability to interrupt or bypass the flow of blood through the chambers of the heart, and thereby directly view the pathology, it was an era of blind or tactile surgery.

The first valve to be approached surgically was the pulmonary valve (between the right ventricle and pulmonary artery). This stemmed from the attention brought to the right ventricular outlet as part of the tetralogy of Fallot. The first successful operation on the pulmonary valve was performed in December 1947 by Sir Thomas Sellors of London. In a twenty-one-year-old man with severe tetralogy of Fallot, a tenotomy knife (similar to that used for cutting tendons) was passed through the right ventricle and the pulmonary valve was incised. The patient improved. In early 1948, Sir Russell Brock carried out a successful transventricular pulmonary valvulotomy, immediately following with two more successes.

The mitral valve attracted more interest because of its relative accessibility and the frequency of lesions. The surgical approaches to pathologic mitral valves were pioneered by three American surgeons, Horace G. Smithy, Jr., Charles P. Bailey, and Dwight E. Harken, and by the British surgeon Sir Russell C. Brock. Each aimed to open the mitral commissures (where the two leaflets of the valve join), usually by a blind and tactile approach to the valve through the atrial appendage, employing a variety of cutting instruments or digital fracture techniques.

Horace G. Smithy Jr. merits primacy for the first truly successful operation on the mitral valve. His obituary in the December 25, 1948, edition of the *Journal of the American Medical Association*, which states that he "is said to have performed the first successful heart valve operation," is not sufficiently assertive. Working in Charleston, South Carolina, Smithy began experimenting on the aortic valve of dogs, probably because he himself was afflicted with severe aortic stenosis (narrowing). He performed eight operations on the mitral valve, excising a segment of the diseased valve and accepting resultant regurgitation. Four of the procedures were carried out through the left ventricle, the other four through the left atrium. The first patient, who was operated upon January 30, 1948, survived only ten months postoperatively and the next two also died shortly after surgery. Subsequently, four patients, including a woman who was operated upon twice, survived for long periods.[29]

Charles P. Bailey of Philadelphia—whose aggressive approach was the subject of mixed reviews, at times extremely critical, and who already had been credited in 1954 with the first successful resection of a ventricular aneurysm resulting from infarction—followed Smithy with an eventually successful mitral commissurotomy (dividing the area where the leaflets of the valve join). After three operative deaths (the first in November 1945), three of five hospitals in Philadelphia withdrew Bailey's privileges. He countered by scheduling two operations to be performed on the same day at two other hospitals. Bailey's first patient died during the operation and he immediately proceeded to Episcopal Hospital, where he successfully cut the lateral commissure of the mitral valve with a knife passed alongside his finger into the atrial appendage. The operation was performed on June 10, 1948, and the patient survived thirty-eight years.[30]

Dwight E. Harken of Peter Bent Brigham Hospital of Boston completed the American troika of surgeons advancing the field of mitral valve surgery. Using a modification of the valvulotome, which Eliot Cutler had employed at the same hospital in 1923, Harken performed his first operation on the mitral valve in March 1947, but the patient died shortly after the procedure. Harken's first success followed Bailey's by six days. Subsequently, through the atrial appendage, Harken incised the mitral commissures of ten patients; six of them died.[31] He then went on to achieve consistent success by dividing the commisssures with his finger or an instrument and dilating the opening of the valve.[32] In England, Russell C. Brock achieved his first success in September 1948 and championed the use of finger fracture of the valve as had been initially proposed by Sir Henry S. Souttar, completing a circular journey of twenty-three years. Elliot Cutler, who first operated on the mitral valve, died in 1947, not living to witness the ultimate success.

Closed repair of narrowing of the aortic valve was more complex and the results did not match the success associated with operations for mitral narrowing. In March 1950, Charles Bailey passed a dilating instrument through a stab wound in the left ventricle to open a stenotic aortic valve. The patient died. As usual, the undaunted Bailey continued on his quest and operated on eleven patients over the next two years. One-third died, but some of the survivors did achieve improvement. He next created a pouch of pericardium, which was sewn to the aorta, thereby permitting direct palpation of the valve and tactile guidance of a dilator. By 1956, Bailey had performed 256 aortic valvulotomies; 40 percent had concomitant mitral valvulotomies.[33] The mortality rate was high. Consistent success awaited the capability of operating on a heart devoid of blood, thereby permitting direct vision of the defect and repair.

Operations for regurgitation through either the mitral or aortic valves also were performed infrequently during this period. They incorporated inventive techniques and generally were associated with less than satisfactory results. Once again, the names of Charles P. Bailey and Dwight E. Harken dominated the field. Bailey used a strip of pericardium passed back and forth through the ventricle, incorporating the base of the mitral septal leaflet to narrow the orifice. This transventricular sling was used in seventy-two patients by Bailey's group during the early 1950s with a 38.5 percent mortality.[34] Bailey's modifications eventually reduced the mortality rate to 16 percent, but the results were not completely satisfying in the survivors. Bailey's accomplishments and the criticisms directed at him were brought into focus by his appearance on the cover of the March 25, 1957, issue of *Time* and an accompanying journalistic narrative.

Dwight E. Harken and his associates were not far behind, and by this time he and Bailey were openly feuding like two matadors vying for supremacy. Initially, Harken's group inserted a Lucite ball in a cage through the atrial appendage and positioned it with transventricular sutures in the heart muscle immediately below the valve. The results were disastrous. Modifications of the prosthesis by using a bottle-shaped or spindle-shaped Lucite prosthesis improved the outcomes, but only minimally.

The surgical treatment of aortic regurgitation was dominated by the ingenuity of Charles Hufnagel, working at Georgetown University. A methyl methacrylate cylinder containing a ball and a cage with a one-way valve was implanted in the descending thoracic aorta of patients. The aorta was cross clamped for about three minutes during which time it was transected, with the prosthesis then quickly being inserted and fixed with two multiple-point nylon rings. The first clinical application took place in September 1952. The favorable result prompted continuance of the application with reasonable short-term results. The clicking of the ball was readily audible when patients opened their mouths, creating an atmosphere of awe during postoperative rounds.[35]

At the same time that blind procedures were performed on the valves of beating, blood-filled hearts, surgical ingenuity was directed at closing intracardiac septal defects, which allowed admixture between blood from the right and the left chambers while maintaining the circulation. In January 1952, Charles P. Bailey performed the first successful repair of the septum between the right and the left atria and later reported fourteen patients with a mortality rate of 14 percent. He inserted his finger through the right atrial appendage to define the defect and guide sutures in order to sew the right atrial wall to the rim of the defect.[36] Robert E. Gross attached a rubber well to the right atrial wall. When the wall was opened, the blood filled the well to the 10 to

12 cm level (i.e., intra-atrial pressure) but did not overflow, allowing the insertion of a finger to guide sutures to repair the defect. Success was first achieved in April 1952.[37]

At the midpoint of the twentieth century, the inability to operate on a bloodless heart and repair defects and diseased valves under direct vision persisted. Three years later, cardiopulmonary bypass would be applied successfully to repair a cardiac lesion for the first time. During the hiatus, two technical innovations allowed surgeons at the University of Minnesota to be the first to repair congenital intracardiac defects while their vision was unimpeded by a bloody field. These innovations, total-body hypothermia and cross circulation, had a short life span but represented important historic bridges.

In the late 1940s, Richard Varco at the University of Minnesota was the first to successfully employ total cardiac inflow occlusion in normothermic patients. He sequentially cross-clamped the superior and inferior vena cavae, allowed six to twelve heartbeats to empty the heart, clamped the pulmonary artery, opened the pulmonary artery proximally, rapidly incised the stenotic pulmonary valve, placed a side clamp on the opening in the artery, released the caval occlusion, and closed the opening in the artery with sutures.

Deep hypothermia would allow for extension of the time during which no blood circulated through the heart and, most important, to the brain. Wilfred P. Bigelow of Toronto produced experimental observations in 1950 that stimulated the use of total-body hypothermia to extend the time that circulation could be interrupted to allow correction of intracardiac defects under direct vision.

In September 1952, F. John Lewis and Mansur Taufic at the University of Minnesota were the first to achieve clinical success with the application of total-body hypothermia to cardiac surgery. By placing the anesthetized patient into a tub full of ice, they reduced the body temperature of a debilitated five-year-old girl to 28 degrees Celsius (82.5 degrees Fahrenheit), allowing the surgeons five and a half minutes of operating time in an empty, bloodless heart to directly repair an atrial septal defect. Henry Swan of Denver, Colorado, followed with three survivors out of four patients. Hypothermia was also used to repair infundibular (muscle beneath the valve) pulmonary valvular stenosis and ventricular septal defects.[38]

Another stopgap that would permit operating within a bloodless heart was developed at the University of Minnesota before mechanical pump oxygenation was universally accepted. The technique, which many have regarded as one of the most courageous and dramatic interventions in the history of cardiac surgery, was human cross-circulation, and the central surgical figure was C. Walton Lillehei. On March 26, 1954, the first procedure was performed on a one-year-old boy with the father as the donor. The blood was removed from the child via a catheter inserted through the jugular vein to provide superior and inferior vena caval drainage, and then pumped into the father's femoral venous system. After circulation through the father's venous system to the lungs where the blood was oxygenated and the carbon dioxide removed, it was returned as arterial blood from the father's femoral artery to the infant's carotid artery to maintain the flow of oxygenated blood to the brain of the

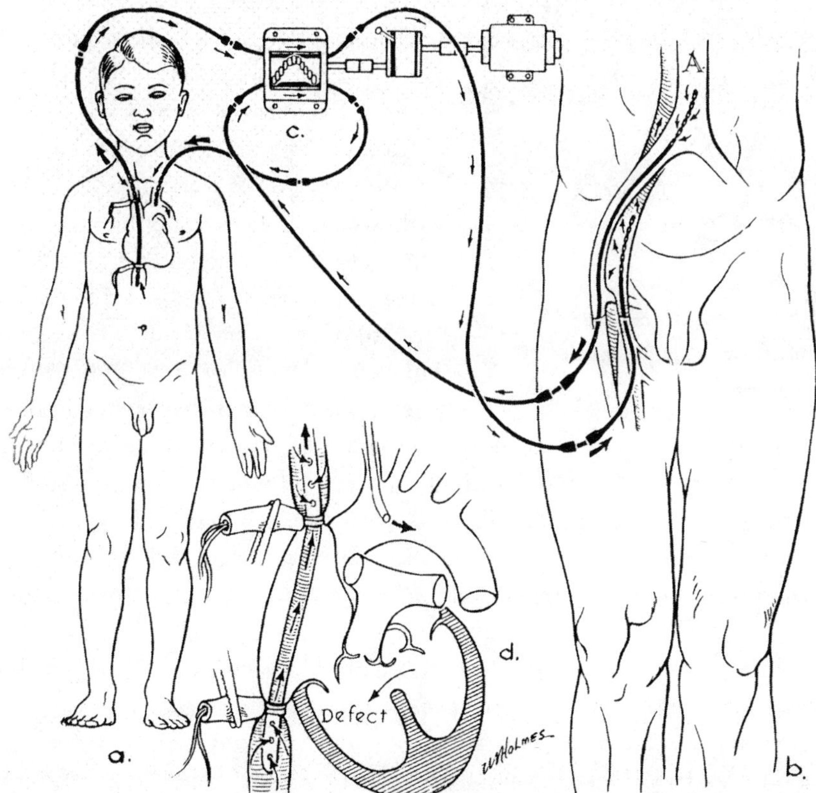

Figure 35: Cross Circulation. C. Walton Lillehei et al., "The Results of Direct Vision Closure of Venticular Septal Defects in Eight Patients by Means of Controlled Cross Circulation," *Surgery, Gynecology & Obstetrics* 101 (1955): 447. Courtesy American College of Surgeons.

child (fig. 35). During the period of cross-circulation, a ventricular defect was repaired but the patient failed to survive. A month later success was achieved when a ventricular septal defect was closed in a four-year-old. Of the forty-five patients who underwent the cross-circulation procedure at the University of Minnesota, twenty-eight survived. No deaths were attributable to the cross-circulation and there was no donor mortality.[39]

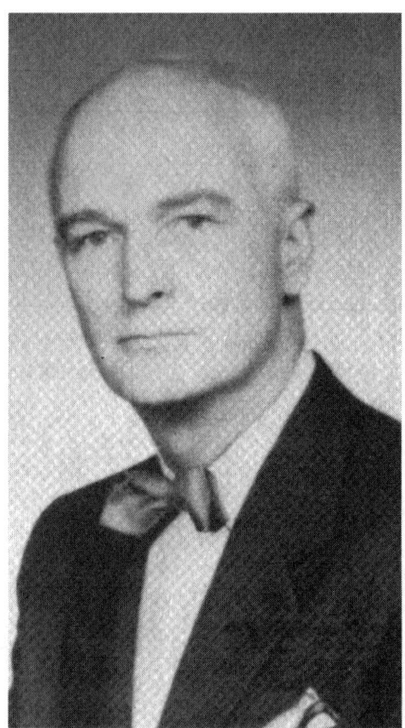
Figure 36: John H. Gibbon Jr. Courtesy of the Archives & Special Collections, Thomas Jefferson University, Philadelphia, Pennsylvania.

The development of a reliable mechanical pump oxygenator unquestionably represents the critical watershed of cardiac surgery; it is the sine qua non that allowed the exciting evolution that has occurred over the past fifty years. The hero, whose dogged determination and ultimately successful quest transformed cardiac surgery, was John H. Gibbon Jr. (fig. 36) of Jefferson Medical College in Philadelphia. The saga of Gibbon's persistent efforts extends over two decades.

Gibbon's quest commenced in 1931 while, as a surgical fellow at Massachusetts General Hospital, he cared for a patient who was dying of a pulmonary embolus. He reasoned that if such a patient's venous blood, which was impeded in its passage through the lung, could be continuously withdrawn into an apparatus that would allow that blood to pick up oxygen and discharge carbon dioxide and then return to the arterial circulation, the patient's condition would improve. Also, the procedure would support the patient's circulation during removal of a pulmonary embolus.[40]

A year later Gibbon and his wife, Maly, who participated throughout all phases of experimentation and development of the heart-lung machine, moved back to Philadelphia. In 1934, the Gibbons returned to Boston for a year to continue their work in the Bullfinch Building at Massachusetts General Hospital and began to develop a machine. The initial problem that Gibbon addressed was the development of a blood oxygenator. The first solution consisted of a vertical revolving cylinder in which the centrifugal force maintained the blood on the inner surface of the cylinder where the blood was exposed to 95 percent oxygen and 5 percent carbon dioxide. The experiments were performed on cats that were often found by the husband and wife researchers in the back alleys of Boston. During those experiments, it was demonstrated that the animals could tolerate thirty to forty minutes of complete extracorporeal bypass of the heart and lungs and that the animals' normal circulation could then be reinstituted.

The results of the experiments conducted in Boston were not completely satisfying and John Gibbon returned to Philadelphia, where he redesigned his machine. One of the modifications was the incorporation of two roller pumps that had been designed by Michael DeBakey in 1934. Gibbon's quest for a heart-lung machine was interrupted by service in World War II. Shortly after he returned to Jefferson Medical College as professor of surgery, he reinstituted efforts to modify the pump oxygenator. IBM engineers assisted him and built sequential models at IBM's Endicott Research Laboratory. The final modification was the oxygenator, which consisted of six flat stainless steel screens enclosed in a plastic case (fig. 37).

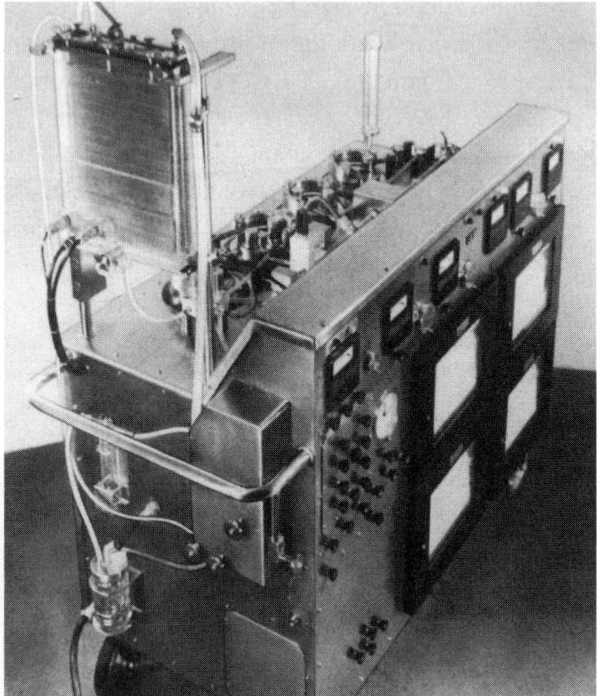

Figure 37: Gibbon's heart-lung machine, model II, 1951. Courtesy of the Archives & Special Collections, Thomas Jefferson University, Philadelphia, Pennsylvania.

John Gibbon's first clinical venture with his heart-lung machine was on a fifteen-month-old girl who died soon after the operation. But the next intervention spelled success. On May 6, 1953, Gibbon closed an atrial septal defect in an eighteen-year-old girl. Complete closure was confirmed by cardiac catheterization months after the procedure. This landmark case constituted the first successful human cardiac operation in which a bloodless field was achieved by means of a heart-lung machine. Two months later Gibbons operated on two more patients; both, however, died. Gibbon was discouraged and thus ended his nineteen-year association with the innovation that revolutionized cardiac surgery. John Gibbon spent the remainder of his career as the Samuel D. Gross Professor of Surgery and chairman of the department of surgery at Jefferson Medical College, where he concentrated on noncardiac thoracic surgery.[41]

John Kirklin, at the Mayo Clinic in Rochester, Minnesota, recognized the importance of what had been accomplished in Philadelphia. He improved Gibbon's machine and applied it with great success, thereby ensuring the permanence of the application of extracorporeal circulation as the basis for the future of cardiac surgery.[42]

Other surgical groups joined the crusade for a reliable heart-lung machine. In 1946, Clarence Crafoord working in Stockholm, Sweden, designed the first such machine to use a rotating disk oxygenator. Most of the experimental work was performed by Viking Björk. At the University of Minnesota, Clarence Dennis began his experiments in the late 1940s. Working with Karl Karlson and others, the group eventually developed a heart-lung machine with multiple, rotating disk screens to provide oxygenation of the blood. On April 5, 1951, two years before John Gibbon's successful procedure, the Minnesota surgeons used their machine and operated on a fifteen-month-old girl with an atrial septal defect. The extracoporeal circulation functioned well, but the patient did not survive.[43]

C. Walton Lillehei energized a continued interest in cardiac surgery at the University of Minnesota. Under his aegis, Richard DeWall developed a functional bubble oxygenator that Lillehei first applied to a patient with success in May 1955. By early 1956, the machine was used in 175 patients undergoing open-heart surgery.[44] The relative simplicity, disposability, and reduced cost of the bubble oxygenator temporarily led to the spread of its use to other centers. But, in the long run, modifications of the Gibbon machine gained permanence.

The mass production of reliable heart-lung machines opened the floodgates for advances in cardiac surgery. Congenital defects were directly repaired, replacing the palliative procedures of the past. The most complex abnormalities responded to surgical ingenuity and operations were performed on newborns and premature infants with success. American surgeons played a leadership role throughout the evolution of these procedures.

Similarly, establishment of a nonbeating, bloodless heart allowed for more-deliberate correction of valvular defects and also the liberal application of coronary artery bypass procedures, once again led by American surgeons. After initial varied attempts to surgically modify diseased valves, attention was directed to the development of prosthetic valves. The first excision and replacement of the mitral valve with a prosthesis was performed in March 1960 at the National Institutes of Health by Nina Braunwald and Andrew Morrow.[45] The patient died sixty hours after completion of the operation, but their second patient, who was operated on the following day, made an uneventful recovery.

Also in 1960, Albert Starr and engineer Miles Lowell Edwards of Portland, Oregon, inserted their first caged ball–valve prosthesis as a replacement for the mitral valve.[46] After several modifications, the device gained broad acceptance. When turned upside down, it was used for aortic valve replacement. Innumerable prosthetic valves of various designs were manufactured and employed, but the Starr-Edwards valve enjoyed the greatest popularity for years, later challenged by the development of porcine preserved homograft valves and tilting disk prostheses.

Advances in surgery for coronary artery occlusion occurred about the same time. The initial approach was thromboendarterectomy (removal of the inner core to widen the conduit blood vessel), and the first successes were reported by Charles Bailey in 1957.[47] Shortly thereafter, Jack Cannon and William P. Longmire Jr. at the University of California, Los Angeles, championed its application in the management of angina pectoris (the pain in the chest associated with coronary artery occlusion).[48] In 1962, David C. Sabiston Jr. at Johns Hopkins was the first to employ aortocoronary bypass with an end-to-end anastomosis between the saphenous vein (taken from the subcutaneous region of the thigh) and the right coronary artery; the patient died three days later of cerebral complications.[49] But it was René Favaloro, an Argentinian working at the Cleveland Clinic, and Dudley Johnson in Milwaukee, Wisconsin, who developed and championed the current technique of coronary artery bypass that resulted in great clinical success and universal acceptance.[50]

The conjoined efforts of surgeons and engineers that led to the development of the heart-lung machine also resulted in the perfection of mechanical devices to assist the failing heart. The first experiments that focused on ventricular assist devices were reported in 1958 by pathologist Bert Kusserow at the University of Vermont. He and his associates developed a motor-driven pump that was placed intra-abdominally in a dog to assist with right and also left ventricular function. He also introduced the transthoracic transfer of energy. The first clinical application of the left ventricular assist device (LVAD) is credited to Hall, DeBakey, and associates, who, in 1963, inserted an artificial left ventricle into the left thorax and established a connection between the left atrium and the descending thoracic aorta. Circulation was maintained for four days.[51]

Michael DeBakey and his associates at Baylor Medical Center evidenced early enthusiasm for the mechanical assistance of cardiac function. In 1971, DeBakey reported his early experience with a left ventricular bypass pump. The first assist device was used in 1963 when it was observed that the heart failed after an aortic valve replacement. Improvement was noted but the patient did not survive. The second patient, who also could not be weaned from cardiopulmonary bypass, was treated with ventricular assistance for ten days and made a complete recovery, the first clinical success using this technology.

Other landmark events in the development of LVAD include the first use of temporary LVAD for postcardiotomy failure in the 1970s, the first use of the device as a bridge to heart transplantation by John Norman, Denton Cooley, and associates at the Texas Heart Institute in Houston in 1978, and the first use of an untethered implantable LVAD as outpatient support by Oscar Frazier in 1994.[52]

The penultimate cardiac surgical feat was the successful transplantation of the human heart, the success of which will be chronicled in the next chapter. The ultimate, as yet unrealized engineering feat related to the heart is the development of an artificial heart. In April 1969, Denton Cooley implanted a total artificial heart for the first time, which had been engineered by Domingo Liotta. The patient regained consciousness after the procedure. The device sustained the circulation for sixty-four hours before transplantation of an allogeneic heart was performed. The patient died thirty-two hours after transplantation. Cooley utilized another artificial heart in July 1981.The patient underwent transplantation, following six hours of mechanical support, and died ten days after that procedure.

In December 1982, William DeVries at the University of Utah for the first time deliberately used an artificial heart, the Jarvik-7 model, as a permanent replacement for a damaged human heart. While the patient died of septicemia 112 days after the operation, the device had functioned well. DeVries and associates operated on three additional patients. One lived, albeit with multiple complications, for more than two years.[53] By 1990, William Pierce of Penn State Medical Center reported that an artificial heart had been inserted in eighty-eight patients as a bridge to cardiac transplantation. Twenty patients died before transplantation. Of the sixty-eight who received a transplant, thirty-three were living at the time of the report.[54]

Advances in cardiac surgery continue with accelerated speed. Robotic techniques, which are being refined, have already allowed for operations on heart valves using minimally invasive techniques that avoid a large incision in the chest wall. The result is less postoperative morbidity and a shortened hospital stay. Endovascular techniques have been used to pass instruments from an artery in the arm or leg to repair or replace the aortic valve. The future of cardiac surgery is almost limitless.

CHAPTER 11:

FROM ONE TO ANOTHER: ORGAN TRANSPLANTATION

The only gift is a portion of thyself.

—Ralph Waldo Emerson
"Gifts" (1844)

In general, surgical success has extended the life of many patients who were doomed to die. The effect of a successful organ transplant, however, is an even more readily apparent change in the recipient's life. It is analogous to the change in an infant following the surgical correction of the tetrology of Fallot, where the infant's color shifts from cyanotic blue to healthy pink. Indeed, the first legendary description of a transplant, attributed to Saints Cosmas and Damian, was characterized by a distinct color change. This prescient legend also involved a set of twins, as would the inception of modern organ transplantation in the scientific era.

The history of organ transplantation has evolved from one organ to another in a series of highly dramatic events. This history invariably begins with such an event that is said to have taken place in the latter half of the third century of the Christian era, involving the twin physicians Cosmas and Damian, who practiced the healing arts in the region of the Gulf of Iskanderum and in the Roman province of Syria. This event was the twins' most famous medical exploit, whereby they successfully grafted the leg of a recently deceased black Ethiopian, whom they exhumed, to replace the ulcerated leg of a Caucasian patient.

Unfortunately, despite their medical prowess, the twins were beheaded circa 303 CE because they refused to recant their Christianity during a time of Roman persecution. The twins became regarded as martyrs and were venerated as saints in the Roman Catholic, the Eastern Orthodox, and the Oriental Orthodox churches. They are considered to be patron saints for all surgeons and physicians.

The modern history of organ transplantation is equally dramatic and associated with towering surgical figures in the United States. This history is most conveniently chronicled according to the individual organs of kidney, pancreas, liver, intestine, and heart and lung.

KIDNEY

The transplantation of the kidney represents the first of four acts in the drama of a donor organ becoming functional in a recipient. Early in the twentieth century, Alexis Carrel conducted a series of experiments on animals in which various organs were successfully transplanted. His contributions have been detailed earlier, where it was noted that in 1912 he received the Nobel Prize in Physiology or Medicine for his work on "vascular anastomosis and transplantation of vessels and organs."

Sporadic, unsuccessful attempts at renal (kidney) transplantation in humans by using pig, sheep, goat, and subhuman primate donors were made by surgeons in France and Germany during the first quarter of the twentieth century. At that time, there was no appreciation of the critical importance of tissue compatibility between donor and recipient. Nor was there any knowledge of the immunologic mechanism that resulted in the rejection of transplanted allogeneic (from one individual to another in the same species) tissues and organs.

In 1936, the Ukranian surgeon Yuriy Yurievich Voronoy reported the first human renal transplant using a human cadaver as the source. The donor kidney's blood vessels were sewn to the femoral vessels in the leg of the recipient and produced urine for two days—on the third day, however, the patient died.[1] Richard Lawler and associates were the first to report the placement of a cadaveric renal transplant within the abdomen.[2] They noted temporary clinical improvement in the uremic patient, but the transplant ceased to function in seven months as a result of rejection. In 1951, eight failed attempts at renal transplantation were reported from France.[3]

Effective organ transplantation required an appreciation of the role of tissue incompatibility between donors and nonidentical twin recipients as the cause for the rejection of the donor organ. Peter B. Medawar, working initially at the Glasgow Royal Infirmary and then in Oxford, England, in the 1950s, is credited with laying the foundation for an appreciation of the immunologic basis of allograft rejection. Tom Gibson, a Scottish surgeon, and Medawar demonstrated that a second skin allograft from the same donor was rejected more rapidly than the first, indicative of an immunologic reaction.[4] It is of interest to note that Medawar's concept of an antibody-mediated cause of skin allograft rejection had been considered by two American investigators decades earlier.

In 1914, H. L. Underwood published in the *Journal of the American Medical Association* observations on skin grafts transplanted sequentially to a burnt patient. The grafts initially survived but later "melted" with later grafts failing more rapidly. In 1924, Emil Holman of San Francisco reported on pinch-skin grafts from a mother to a child. After early complete coverage of the outer layer, the patient developed widespread dermatitis that responded to removal of the grafts. Holman stated: "It occurred to me that the general dermatitis was most probably a phenomenon of anaphylaxis or protein intoxication, and a manifestation of sensitiveness to a foreign protein." Medawar was aware of these publications when he began his own investigations into the matter.[5]

Successful renal transplantation was first achieved in 1954 at Peter Bent Brigham Hospital in Boston as the result of a carefully executed plan to develop the specific transplantation of this organ. Dr. George Thorn, the physician-in-chief at that hospital, established a program to treat end-stage renal disease shortly after the conclusion of World War II. The dialysis machine that was developed in Holland by Willem Kolff was modified by staff physicians at Peter Bent Brigham Hospital and the first dialysis program in the United States was established there. In 1948, Francis D. Moore, the newly appointed surgeon-in-chief, added his enthusiastic support. A multidisciplinary unit involving physicians and surgeons was created to further explore renal transplantation and it became a major focus of the hospital.

The first surgeon to participate in the program was a general surgeon, David M. Hume, who was joined by Joseph E. Murray, a plastic surgeon (fig. 38). The surgical investigators successfully autotransplanted the kidneys of dogs, who survived with normal renal function for long periods of time, proving that interruption of the nerve supply of the kidney did not impede the filtering effect of the organ or the production of adequate urine. During the course of those experiments, they also determined the optimal site for placement of a donor kidney in the pelvis.

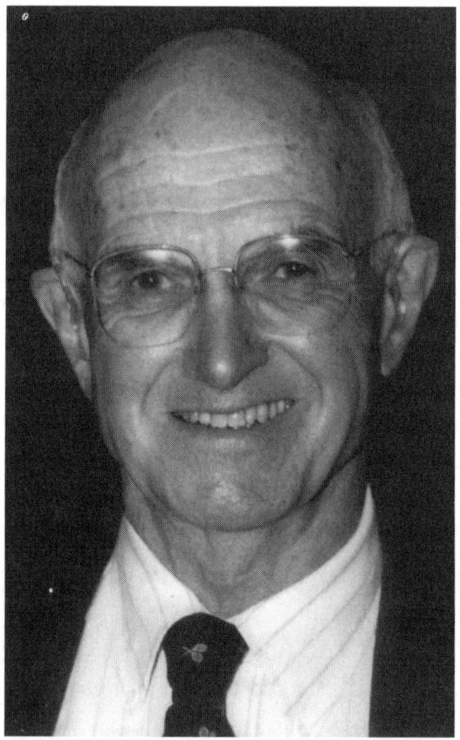

Figure 38: Joseph E. Murray. Courtesy of Joseph E. Murray.

Between April 1951 and December 1952, Hume transplanted eight cadaver kidneys into the thighs of nonimmunosuppressed patients with renal failure after he had previously transplanted one kidney into the normal location. One graft, which was positioned in the thigh, produced urine for nine months. With the rest of the grafts suffering rejection, the other seven recipients' course provided a classic description of renal allograft rejection in subjects not receiving immunosuppressive therapy.[6] Hume's one long-term functioning renal transplant in a nonimmunosuppressed individual, however, was cited by Thomas Starzl a half century later as support for the potential of preoperative desensitization of recipients to minimize incompatibility.

The first successful renal transplant involved identical twins. It took place, in part, because of a Massachusetts physician's awareness that the staff of Peter Bent Brigham Hospital was currently engaged in research focused on renal transplantation. The Massachusetts physician, Dr. David C. Miller of the US Public Health Service, was caring for Richard Herrick, a patient whose health was rapidly deteriorating because of kidney failure. Miller perceptively recognized the potential that Richard's identical twin, Ronald—with an identical genetic composition—represented a unique source for a kidney that could sustain Richard's life. Therefore, the patient was referred to Peter Bent Brigham Hospital in October 1954, specifically with renal transplantation in mind.

The patient's preoperative status was improved by using dialysis. Ethical and psychiatric issues were discussed extensively because it was the first time in history that a normal person was being subjected to a major surgical operation with its attendant risk for the sole benefit of another. Extrapolating from Peter Medawar's classical experiments, surgeons transferred a skin graft from Ronald to Richard, which demonstrated no sign of rejection. This provided the strongest evidence of genetic identity and the absence of any immunologic barrier that would lead to rejection of tissue or organ, a circumstance that had been defined previously by the plastic surgeon James Barrett Brown in 1957.[7]

On December 23, 1954, J. Hartwell Harrison, the professor of urology at Peter Bent Brigham Hospital, removed Ronald's donor kidney, which was then transported by Francis D. Moore to an adjacent room where it was implanted into Richard by Joseph E. Murray. Dr. Murray had replaced Hume as codirector with John P. Merrill of the transplant program when Hume left to serve as a medical officer during the Korean War.

Almost immediately after the clamps were removed from the arteries and veins that attached the donor kidney to the recipient's circulation, blood flowed smoothly to and from the transplanted kidney, while urine flowed from the ureter before it was implanted into the bladder.[8] Richard had his own two kidneys removed at two subsequent operations that were performed within the ensuing six months. He survived eight years after the transplant at which time he died from recurrence of the original disease, chronic nephritis, in the transplanted kidney. The Brigham group continued to perform renal transplants in identical twins and, three years after the first case had been reported, Murray and associates published the successful results of six additional renal transplantations between identical twins.[9]

The aim was to expand the pool of candidates for renal transplants beyond that of identical twins by preventing rejection of the transplanted kidney that occurred because of immunologic incompatibility of nonidentical twins or unrelated donors. The first approach consisted of total-body irradiation to ablate the recipient's immune system by destroying the immune cells within the bone marrow and lymph nodes. Once the transplant was functional, marrow cells were introduced by infusion. This protocol was first applied clinically by the Brigham group in 1957. Both patients so treated died one month after the procedure because of lack of marrow function and widespread infection.

Sublethal irradiation without marrow transfusion was employed in the next ten patients. All but one died within one month of the renal transplantation. One patient, who had received a kidney from his fraternal twin, survived with good renal function for twenty years, representing the first example of a successful transplant in the face of a genetic barrier.[10]

The failure associated with marrow irradiation provoked a search for pharmacologic immunosuppression. On April 5, 1962, Joseph Murray performed the first successful cadaver kidney transplant in which immunosuppression, using azathioprine (Imuran), was achieved and long-term success resulted.[11] The results, however, remained suboptimal until Thomas Starzl and associates at the University of Colorado coupled the administration of smaller doses of azathioprine with prednisone.[12] Subsequently, good results were consistently reported. Therapeutic regimens, in which the dosages of the immunosuppresive drugs were reduced, lessened the toxic effects and improved the posttransplant patient's general well-being while also maintaining renal function.

Once pharmacologic immunosuppression became available, clinical xenotransplantation (from one species to another) of kidneys from chimpanzees by Keith Reemtsma in New Orleans and from baboons by Thomas Starzl in Colorado captured the headlines in the media. The results, however, were uniformly unsatisfactory.

Nonetheless, the introduction of the immunosuppressives cyclosporine and tacrolimus had dramatic effects and provided significantly improved management of patients receiving grafts from unrelated human donors, thus allowing renal transplantation to become an integral service in most academic medical centers.

In 1990, Joseph E. Murray shared the Nobel Prize for Physiology or Medicine with E. Donnall Thomas for "their discoveries concerning organ and cell transplantation." Murray became the third surgical recipient of that prize for work performed in the United States, following Alexis Carrel in 1912 and Charles Brenton Huggins, a urologist at the University of Chicago who was recognized in 1966 "for his discoveries concerning the hormonal treatment of prostatic cancer." Since Alexis Carrel was French and Charles Huggins was born in Canada, Joseph E. Murray was the first surgeon who was a native citizen of the United States to be so honored.

PANCREAS

When compared with the kidney, transplantation of the pancreas is a significantly less frequent procedure. In most instances with pancreas transplants, the organ has been transplanted either simultaneously with or after a kidney transplant. Infrequently, isolated transplantation of the pancreas has been performed for diabetes mellitus. One of the morbid complications of diabetes mellitus, particularly type 1 and insulin-dependent type 2, relates to renal failure. At the onset of the era of renal transplantation, diabetes mellitus was considered a contraindication (a condition that greatly increases risk) to the procedure. In the course of time, however, patients with diabetes mellitus became acceptable candidates for renal transplantation. Ultimately, attention was directed at correcting the metabolic disorder associated with diabetes, which caused the renal pathology that led to renal failure. Transplantation of the pancreas or of isolated islet cells offered a potential solution.

In 1957, Irving Lichtenstein, who would later achieve eponymic fame for his tension-free repair of inguinal (groin) hernias, and Richard Barshak of Los Angeles published the first description of intra-abdominal transplantation of the pancreas using vascular anastomosis in dogs. But there was no measurement of glucose levels or insulin production postoperatively in the experimental animals, and no viable pancreatic tissue remained at the graft site six weeks after the procedure.[13] Keith Reemtsma and his associates at Tulane University in New Orleans were the first to report temporary function of pancreatic transplants in dogs, who had their own pancreas removed. Viability of the graft lasted for up to ten days, as evidenced by a lowering of the blood sugar, before rejection occurred.[14]

Clinical transplantation of the pancreas in humans had its genesis at the University of Minnesota on December 17, 1966. William Kelly, with the assistance of Richard C. Lillehei, transplanted a segmental pancreas graft in which the pancreatic duct was ligated. The pancreas transplant was performed simultaneously with a kidney transplant in an insulin-dependent, type 1 diabetic recipient. The patient remained insulin free for six days, at which point she again required insulin. Two months after the original operation, she developed pancreatitis in the graft, necessitating removal of both the pancreas and the rejected kidney. She died thirteen days after the second operation.[15]

Between 1966 and 1973, Richard C. Lillehei performed twelve more pancreas transplants. The technique was modified to a transplantation of the whole organ. In eight instances a concomitant renal transplant was performed; in four cases only the pancreas was transplanted. Rejection was a frequent event. One encouraging result occurred in a patient with a pancreas-kidney transplant, who sustained a functional pancreas for almost one year.[16]

In 1969, Fred Merkel and Thomas Starzl at the University of Colorado and also John Connolly and associates at Stanford each performed one partial pancreas-kidney transplant. The first pancreas transplant that was performed outside the United States was not carried out until 1972. In November 1971, Marvin Gliedman at Montefiore Hospital and Medical Center in the Bronx, New York, performed the first pancreas transplant in which the pancreatic duct was drained into the recipient's ureter (urinary tract).[17] Gliedman's group went on to perform eleven such procedures and reported one graft that functioned for twenty-two months and another for fifty months.[18]

In 1983, Hans Sollinger at the University of Wisconsin introduced the technique for providing pancreatic ductal drainage directly into the bladder.[19] The next year, Starzl and associates reintroduced and championed draining the ducts into the intestine, thereby maintaining the natural course for pancreatic juice.[20] This technique is currently the most frequently employed. As of 2004, more than twenty-five thousand complete or partial pancreas transplants had been performed throughout the world.[21]

An attractive alternative to partial or whole organ pancreas transplantation is injection of sufficient amounts of donor islet cells that produce insulin and that sustain their control of the glucose level. In 1967, Paul Lacy and Mery Kostianovsky at Washington University in St. Louis reported a method for isolating islets of Langerhans (the cells that produce insulin) from the rat pancreas.[22] R.Younozai and associates performed the first transplantation of isolated islet cells from one animal to another two years later.[23] Their work was followed by that of Walter Ballinger and Paul Lacy, who demonstrated that the islets respond by increasing insulin production when perfused with high concentrations of glucose. Islet grafts in diabetic immunosuppressed rats reduced the diabetic state.[24]

The first clinical transplantation of isolated pancreatic islets from a donor to a recipient was carried out at the University of Minnesota in 1974, but the graft functioned poorly.[25] In 1980, Felix Largiader and associates in Zurich, Switzerland, were the first to report insulin independence (indicating success of the graft) in a type 1 diabetic patient after an islet transplant.

In 1990, Andreas Tzakis, Starzl, and a group in Pittsburgh reported sparing a child from diabetes who had undergone removal of the liver, pancreas, stomach, and upper abdominal organs followed by liver transplantation, by infusing the donor's purified islet cells into the portal vein of the transplanted liver.[26] Several groups in the United States followed with sporadic successes.[27] The results were significantly improved in 2000 by a group at the University of Alberta, Canada, but, to date, there has been no consistent success.[28]

LIVER

In chronological order, the liver was the second organ to be transplanted in humans. It was the first of the unpaired organs to be transplanted, and, initially, the first to be dependant upon a cadaver donor. In 1969, *Experience in Hepatic Transplantation* was published with over five hundred pages of text that considered all aspects of the subject at a time when the author was able to chronicle only twenty-five human recipients of replacement allografts. A figure depicting the life survival curve of those patients poignantly indicates that all seven of the patients operated on through June 1967 died within the first four weeks, either due to technical surgical accidents or the use of damaged allografts. Among the next nine patients, operated on between July 1967 and May 1968, three were alive at one year, while only one of the nine patients operated on during the subsequent eight months was alive five months after the procedure.[29]

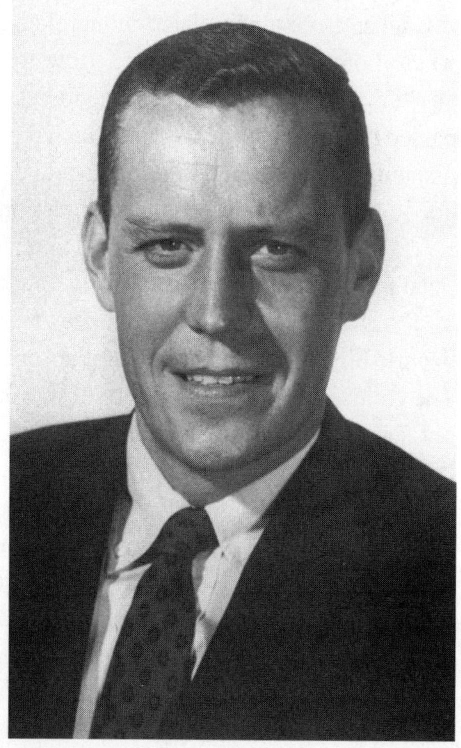

Figure 39: Thomas E. Starzl. Courtesy of Thomas E. Starzl.

The senior surgeon who coauthored the book and whose research and clinical experience formed the basis for the text was Thomas E. Starzl (fig. 39), whose reaction to the discouraging data was one of determination and dogged optimism rather than despondency. His indefatigability and persistence in the face of repeated early failures, pessimism by the medical establishment, and vitriolic attacks by the lay press are legendary. Starzl has achieved iconic stature and is unquestionably recognized as the dominant individual in the birth and development of liver transplantation as an acceptable addition to the surgical armamentarium.

Starzl proved his potential as an inventive leader in medicine while still in medical school. Under the guidance of Horace W. Magoun, Starzl, while a medical student at Northwestern and a graduate student at University of California, Los Angeles, completed seminal work in neuroanatomy. He employed deep recording techniques in the brain to measure electrical responses to sensory stimuli and thereby track the reticular activating system.[30]

While Starzl was still in the midst of his surgical residency in 1955, C. Stuart Welch, the chair of the department of surgery at the Albany Medical College, reported the transplantation of an auxiliary liver in a dog. A donor liver was taken from a nonrelated mongrel and placed within the abdominal cavity, where both arterial and venous flow to the donor liver were established by anastomosis with the recipient blood vessels. The outflow from the donor liver passed into the vena cava, from which it passed to the heart. Although the transplanted livers produced bile for several days, function ceased shortly thereafter due to the absence of immunosuppression, which resulted in rejection.[31]

Preceding the first orthotopic liver transplant, an auxiliary liver transplantation in a human was performed at the University of Minnesota in 1964 by Karel B. Absolon and associates on a thirteen-month-old child with extrahepatic biliary atresia (congenital absence of the bile ducts outside the liver). The child, into whom a donor liver was attached by vascular anastomosis, did not survive.[32] Several other teams, including Starzl's, attempted similar procedures without success.

Starzl's contributions to the initiation and perfection of liver transplantation have extended over the past half century. While he was at the University of Miami between 1956 and 1958, he developed a standard technique for removal of the entire liver of a dog. During these experiments, he realized that this represented the first stage of liver transplantation into its normal location and he presciently visualized a new liver being inserted into the empty space. After he moved to a faculty position at the Northwestern University Medical Center in Chicago in 1958, Starzl began to develop a technique for replacing the liver with a cadaveric donor. The animals manifested temporary functional success, which lasted until rejection inevitably brought about functional failure of the liver and death.

At about the same time that Starzl began his investigations, Francis D. Moore and associates began parallel research at Peter Bent Brigham Hospital. In 1960, this group reported on thirty-one liver transplant experiments in which seven animals lived without immunosuppression for more than four days.[33] In a discussion of that paper, Starzl indicated that he had performed orthotopic liver transplants on eighteen dogs that survived four days, with one living for twenty and a half days. Also in the 1960s, Starzl reported multivisceral organ transplants in dogs, in which the stomach, intestines, and pancreas were transplanted en masse with the liver.[34]

From 1961 through 1980, Starzl's work was carried out at the University of Colorado's Medical Center in Denver. In 1963, after he had established a successful kidney transplantation program, and at a time when the effectiveness of the combination of azathioprine and steroid therapy as an immunosuppression regimen was established for kidneys, Starzl performed the first orthotopic (in its normal location) liver transplant in a human. The patient was a three-year-old child with biliary atresia; the donor was a child who died during an open-heart procedure and was maintained on a heart-lung machine. The transplantation, however, was not completed because the recipient had uncontrollable bleeding. That year four additional liver transplants were performed with no survivors, resulting in a self-imposed moratorium for Starzl, which extended for more than three years.[35]

The next phase in the saga of liver transplantation was initiated by Strazl's report to the American Surgical Association in 1968. This report replaced the sense of doom regarding liver transplantations with a more hopeful outlook. In that report, all seven children who had liver transplants survived the procedure and the thirty-day immediate postoperative period. Four died within six months but three were alive at the time of the report. In the latter group, two died of recurrent cancer about a year later and the remaining patient, operated on for biliary atresia, died two and a half years after the procedure due to chronic rejection.[36]

By February 1969, the Colorado team had performed twenty-six human liver transplants, including one with a chimpanzee donor and a few auxiliary livers. Although six lived for a year, all died as a result of recurrence of cancer or rejection within two and a half years. In 1975, by which time ninety-three cases of liver transplantation had been performed at Colorado, the only other program in the world, directed by Roy Calne in Cambridge, King's College, England, had results that paralleled those of Starzl with but a few long-term survivors.

After a hiatus of about four years, during which time cyclosporine became available and transformed the entire transplant scene by providing effective immunosuppression, Starzl performed a small series of successful liver transplants in Colorado. In 1980, the undaunted surgical pioneer moved east to the University of Pittsburgh Medical Center, which became the Mecca of liver transplantation. The early times in Pittsburgh were hardly halcyon days for Starzl. The first four patients who had liver transplants died within twenty-one days of the operation and the failures evoked cries for cessation of the entire program. But the tide turned and twenty of the next twenty-three liver transplant recipients enjoyed long-term survival. Twenty-six patients received liver transplants in 1981 and the number doubled each year for the ensuing five years.[37] Not only did the procedure gain legitimacy, but the surgeons trained by Starzl spread forth with apostolic zeal throughout the world to transform a clinical experiment into a practical and acceptable clinical surgical procedure.

Emboldened by their success, Starzl and his associates extended their vistas. The development of an effective antirejection regimen allowed the clinical application of the so-called cluster procedure (liver, pancreas, intestines), which Starzl had described in dogs in 1959. This triad was pared down to the liver and intestine. In 1992, the Pittsburgh team was able to report five successful solely small intestinal transplants, following which patients could eat and shed their intravenous feeding tubes.[38]

Perhaps the most publicized of the Pittsburgh operations was the first combined liver-heart transplantation in 1984 on Stormie Jones. The patient was a victim of familial hypercholesterolemia (excessively high levels of blood cholesterol), which was caused by a metabolic malfunction of the liver. The condition is associated with premature atherosclerostic occlusion of arteries throughout the body and, in particular, to the heart, causing myocardial infarction and impaired cardiac function. On St. Valentine's Day 1984, Henry T. Bahnson, the chairman of the department of surgery, performed the heart transplant and two surgeons trained by Starzl sewed in the donor liver. The result was a bipartite success—the heart functioned well and the hypercholesterolemia was corrected by the donor liver.[39] In early 1990, the patient underwent a second liver transplantation but died at the end of the year.

HEART AND LUNG

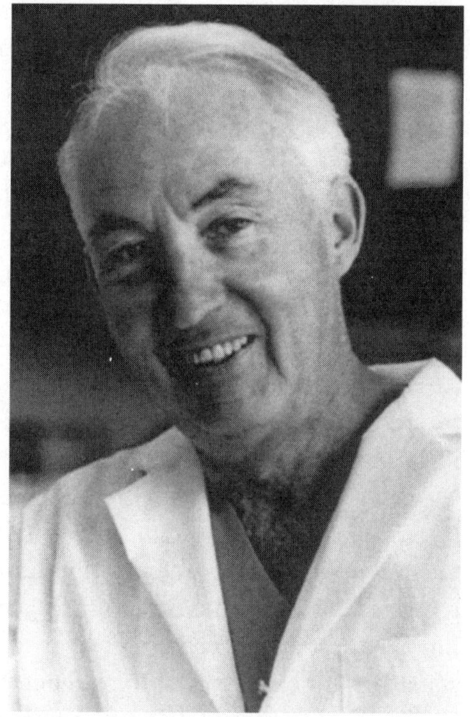

Figure 40: Norman E. Shumway. Courtesy of Sara J. Shumway.

Sir Francis Darwin wrote, "In science credit goes to the man who convinces the world."[40] Christiaan Barnard performed the first heart transplant in a human and there was a time that recognition of his name throughout the world was exceeded only by that of President John F. Kennedy. Norman Edward Shumway (fig. 40), however, is generally awarded the appellation of the Father of Transplantation of the Heart because he initiated the research and developed the technique that eventuated in success. His name joins that of Joseph E. Murray and Thomas E. Starzl as a triumvirate of pioneers in organ transplantation.

As noted earlier, the history of cardiac transplantation was initiated with the experiments of Alexis Carrel and Charles Claude Guthrie in the early part of the twentieth century. Among the many organs to which they applied their newly developed techniques of vascular anastomosis was the donor heart of experimental animals. The donor hearts were transplanted into the neck of each recipient using the cervical blood vessels as the attachments. In one instance, they transplanted the heart and lungs of a kitten into the neck of an adult cat.

In 1933, Frank Mann and his associates at the Mayo Clinic laboratories reported an extension of the work of Carrel and Guthrie after transplanting the heart to the neck and creating a preparation in which only the right side of the heart was functional in dogs. The average survival of those transplanted hearts was four days, although one preparation continued to beat for eight days.[41]

In Russia during the 1940s and 1950s, Vladimir Demikhov conducted a remarkable series of diverse transplant procedures that remained unknown to the Western world until 1962. The most bizarre of these consisted of the transplantation of the heads and limbs of puppies onto the torsos of adult dogs after which function of the donor tissues lasted for as long as twenty-nine days. Among the many organs transplanted by Deminkhov were isolated hearts or hearts combined with a lobe of the lung into the chest of the recipients as auxiliary organs. One dog was sacrificed at thirty-two days. The Russian also performed sixty-seven orthotopic transplants of heart-lung preparations and reported two survivors of up to fifteen hours.[42] In a series of reports, Watts Webb and associates at the University of Mississippi from 1953 through 1968 removed and replaced the dogs' own hearts and also transplanted donor canine hearts with the support of the heart-lung machine.[43]

In 1958, Norman Edward Shumway and Richard Rowland Lower began their experimentation in cardiac transplantation at the Stanford University Medical Center. Four years later, the Stanford group reported the successful transplantation of dog donor hearts after preservation.[44] Shortly thereafter, the group reported suppression of rejection in the cardiac allograft; four dogs remained alive for more than four years. In the course of these studies, Shumway and his associates developed a procedure that would serve as the standard surgical approach throughout the world.[45]

The first transplantation of a heart in a human was reported by James D. Hardy of the University of Mississippi in 1963. Because no human donor organ was available, the heart of a large chimpanzee was transplanted, but it was not able to support the recipient's circulation.[46] A year earlier, Hardy had reported the first case of lung transplantation in a man. The transplanted lung functioned but the patient died eighteen days after the operation from preexisting renal failure.[47]

No medical event was reported with greater worldwide publicity than the orthotopic transplantation of a human donor heart by Christiaan Neethling Barnard into Louis Washkansy on December 3, 1967, at the Groote Schuur Hospital in Capetown, South Africa. The patient died eighteen days after the operation due to a pulmonary infection. The autopsy showed that the transplanted heart had maintained circulation and showed no evidence of rejection.[48] Several physicians and surgeons in the United States were critical of the transplant, considering it premature, labeling the surgeon as "presumptuous." Others, including Norman Shumway, welcomed the remarkable achievement.

The first heart transplant in the United States was performed by Adrian

Kantrowitz at Maimonides Hospital in Brooklyn. Three days after the operation by Barnard, Kantrowitz transplanted the heart from an anencephalic (congenital absence of the brain) infant into a two-day-old baby, who died a few hours after the operation.[49] The race for success was on.

On January 2, 1968, Barnard transplanted a heart into Philip Blaiberg, who lived eighteen months before dying from rejection of the graft, thereby representing the first cardiac transplant with an extended survival. Four days after Blaiberg received a new heart, Shumway entered the clinical competition at Stanford University, but the patient died fifteen days after the procedure following a series of complications. A few months later, Kantrowitz performed his second heart transplant, and Denton Cooley performed his first cardiac transplantation at St. Luke's Hospital in Houston, Texas.

Within a period of six months, Cooley's team performed nine heart transplants, including the use of a sheep's heart in one instance. The first patient in that series, Everett Thomas, represented the first success in the United States. During the year that followed Barnard's groundbreaking procedure, more than one hundred cardiac transplants were performed around the world in more than fifty institutions. Initial enthusiasm was tempered, however, because more than 60 percent of the patients died within eight days and the mean survival time was fewer than thirty days.[50]

In 1975, Barnard was the first to institute a clinical program that transplanted auxiliary hearts to aid the patient's poorly functioning heart, which remained in place. Interest in this procedure faded as a result of Shumway and associates' advances with the replacement procedure. Improvements in technique, logistics related to donations, and immunosuppression spearheaded by the Stanford group resulted in worldwide acceptance of heart transplantation. By 1989, the hospital mortality following the procedure was less than 10 percent and the five-year actuarial survival had increased to almost 75 percent.[51]

The first combined heart-lung transplant was performed by Cooley on a two-and-a-half-year-old in 1969. The patient died within a day. C Walton Lillehei and Barnard also performed the procedure before Bruce Reitz and the Stanford team achieved success in 1981.[52] By 1988, more than two hundred patients received the combined heart-lung transplant, and the one-year actuarial survival was more than 60 percent.

Eventually, all of the surgical pioneers in organ transplantation must have reflected on the naysayers and the hurdles they overcame with a sense of pride in their accomplishments. In 2005, a total of 27,527 organs were transplanted in the United States: 16,072 kidneys, 896 kidney-pancreases, 129 pancreases after kidneys, 129 pancreases alone, 6,000 livers, 68 intestines, 2,063 hearts, 1,405 lungs, and 32 heart-lungs.[53] The success rates are laudable and each of the procedures has gained worldwide acceptance in the care of patients with organ failure.

CHAPTER 12:

SMATTERINGS FROM THE SPECIALTIES

The multitudinous facts presented by each corner of Nature form in large part the scientific man's burden today, and restrict him more willy-nilly, to a narrower and narrower specialism.

—John Newport Langley
Report of the British Association for the Advancement of Science (1899)

In the past, cynics opined that experts and specialists were those who knew more and more about less and less. With the information and technical explosions that have occurred in medicine and surgery during the passage of the twentieth century, it is now more appropriate to characterize a specialist as one who knows more and more about more and more.

In appreciation of the rapid expansion of knowledge, it became necessary to define specialty qualifications and issue certifications that would assure the public of the specialist's possession of those qualifications. In 1908, Derrick T. Vail first proposed in his presidential address to the American Academy of Ophthalmology and Otolaryngology the concept of a specialty board. Despite the fact that academic departments of surgery, which developed in the United States during the early part of the twentieth century, generally included all specialties, by 1933 the boards of Opthalmology, Otolaryngology, Dermatology, and Obstetrics and Gynecology had been formed and joined to establish the Advisory Board for Medical Specialties. The function of this newly created consortium was to oversee the examination and certification of all specialty boards. The American Board of Surgery, which was created in 1937, as well as the American Board of Orthopaedic Surgery (1935), the American Board of Urology (1935), the American Board of Neurological Surgery (1940), the American Board of Plastic Surgery (1941), and the American Board of Colon and Rectal Surgery (1949) followed suit and joined the advisory board.

In 1970, the Advisory Board for Medical Specialties was reorganized to form the American Board of Medical Specialties (ABMS), which by 1971 included the American Board of Thoracic Surgery. These specialty boards became responsible for certifying the special qualifications within each of their designated specialties. The American Board of Surgery, for instance, certifies the special qualifications for pediatric surgery and general vascular surgery.

An arbitrary selection of contributions to the formally recognized areas of surgical specialization offers but a smattering from an extensive list. These contributions do, however, provide added evidence of the panoramic scope of American influence on the evolution of surgery.

OTOLARYNGOLOGY

In otolaryngology one of the early contributions was the modern technique of rhinoplasty. At the beginning of the tweentieth century, John Orlando Roe of Rochester, New York, published the results for his technique of rhinoplasty that became the basis for the current approach and preceded the reports of similar procedures in Europe.[1] When considering the diverse aspects of otolaryngology (the study of the ear, nose, and throat), there are three Americans who are regarded as giants. The names of Chevalier Jackson, Hayes Martin, and William House are, respectively, synonymous with endoscopy, head and neck surgery, and inner ear surgery.

The much-honored Chevalier Jackson, who worked in Pittsburgh and Philadelphia, developed an esophagoscope in 1890 through which he extracted a dental plate from an adult's esophagus and a coin from a child's esophagus. Jackson improved the technique of tracheotomy and essentially invented bronchoscopy, the endoscopic visual investigation of the airway. After he devised his first esophagoscope, he managed many cases of lye burns of the esophagus. As a consequence, he championed the federal Caustic Act of 1927 that mandated every can of lye or other caustic substance to display the word "POISON" in large letters to avoid dangerous errors.[2] Hayes Martin of Memorial Hospital in New York City pioneered the removal of tumors in the oral cavity. His book *Surgery of Head and Neck Tumors* (1957) was the classic textbook covering the subject.[3] The basis for current microlaryngeal removal of vocal cord tumors was the result of Geza J. Jako's pioneering work with the carbon dioxide laser. The first clinical report of its use appeared in 1972.[4] William House of Los Angeles merits recognition as the father of the related subspecialty otoneurology (the neural aspects of the inner ear related to hearing and equilibrium). His contributions span the fields of acoustic tumor surgery, Meniere's disease (a disease manifest by vertigo, ringing in the ear, and deafness), and cochlear implants.[5]

ORTHOPAEDICS

Also emanating from American soil was the advancement of orthopaedics (study of musculoskeletal system). In the 1850s, Gordon Buck at New York Hospital introduced the adhesive-strapping-traction method for treatment of fracture of the femur, which still remains in use.[6] In 1891, Berthold Ernest Hadra, a German immigrant in Texas, published the first report of spinal fusion, using silver wire to fix the spinous processes of the sixth and seventh cervical vertebrae, later applying the technique to tuberculosis of the spine (Pott's disease).[7] Russell Hibbs of New York Orthopaedic Hospital described the first spinal fusion operation using bridging bone grafts, initially for tuberculosis in 1911, and subsequently for scoliosis in 1914.[8] The introduction of the Milwaukee brace by Walter P. Blount and others and the method of internal fixation of Paul Harrington of Houston subsequently were adopted for the treatment of scoliosis.[9]

In 1933, Darryl B. Phemister of Chicago introduced the technique of removing a block from the epiphyseal plate (the area of growth at the end of long bones) to correct abnormal length and angular deformities of the lower extremities.[10] In 1949, Walter P. Blount and George R. Clarke modified this procedure by applying staples to the growth plates.[11] Marius Smith-Peterson of Boston significantly advanced the treatment of hip fractures by inserting a triflanged nail to withstand bending and rotational stress. Initially, this was placed using an incision to visualize the region directly. Later, the nail was inserted with radiological guidance without open exposure.[12] Americans were particularly notable for their leadership role related to surgery of the hand. Allan B. Kanavel's *Infections of the Hand* (1933) and Sterling Bunnell's *Surgery of the Hand* (1944) are both regarded as classics.

UROLOGY

On October 5, 1904, William Stewart Halsted performed the first operation in the new operating room suites at the Johns Hopkins Hospital. The other participants included: as first assistant, James M. T. Finney, who would become professor of surgery at Johns Hopkins and the first president of the American College of Surgeons; as second assistant, Joseph C. Bloodgood, who is credited as the first surgeon to wear rubber surgical gloves and also a future professor of surgery at Johns Hopkins; and Harvey Cushing and Hugh Hampton Young. The photograph of the event has been given the title of the "All-Star Operation."

Hugh Hampton became the first professor of urology at John Hopkins University. His name has been attached to two operations: the perineal prostatectomy (removal of the prostate gland through the region between the scrotum and anus) for benign enlargement and the radical perineal prostatectomy for cancer of the prostate.[13] In the 1980s, Patrick Walsh, also at Johns Hopkins, refined the radical prostatectomy to preserve urinary continence and sexual potency.[14] Eugene M. Bricker, a general surgeon at Washington University in St. Louis, is recognized for his contribution of the ileal conduit in which the ureters are anastomosed to an isolated portion of ileum (distal small intestine), thereby diverting the urine, which empties into a collection bag. This procedure became standard during evisceration of the pelvis in the treatment of bladder and uterine cancers.[15]

American urology also can lay claim to a Nobel laureate. In 1966, Charles B. Huggins (fig. 41) of the University of Chicago received the Nobel Prize in Physiology or Medicine for demonstrating the capability of altering the prognosis of cancer of the prostate by changing the hormonal environment within the patient.

NEUROSURGERY

While Harvey Cushing's central role in the development of the specialty of neurosurgery has been considered in chapter 8, Walter A. Dandy, a towering figure who shared eminence with Cushing, is also worth considering. Dandy began as a research assistant for Cushing at Johns Hopkins in the Hunterian

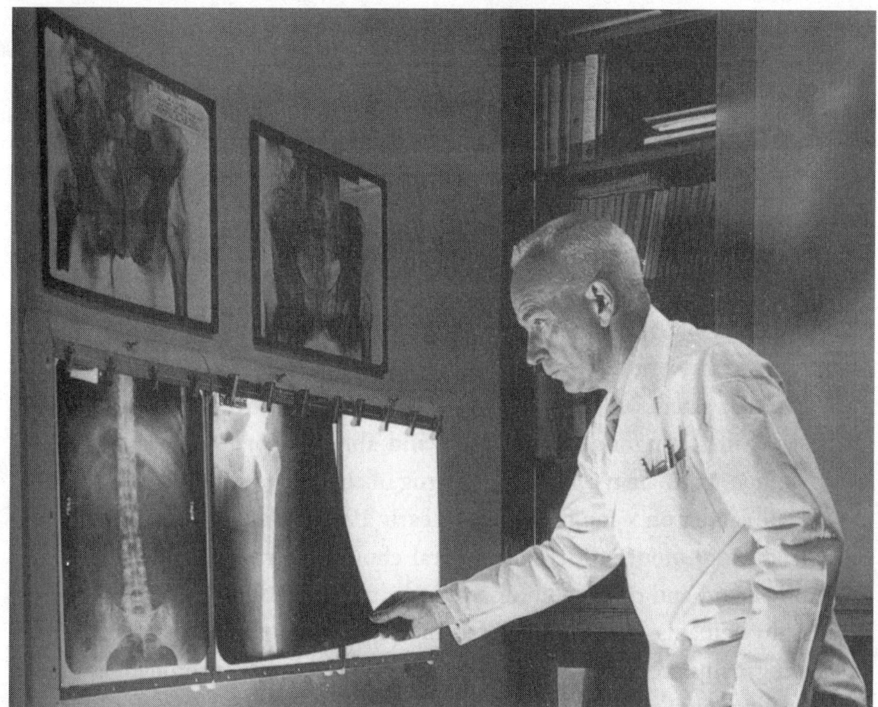

Figure 41: Charles Huggins. Courtesy of Special Collections Research Center, University of Chicago Library.

Laboratory and eventually grew to the status of a major competitor with Cushing. From the onset, the relationship between the two men was strained and only intensified when Cushing elected not to invite Dandy to join him at Peter Bent Brigham Hospital. Therefore, Dandy, whom many regarded as the more facile technical surgeon, assumed the leadership role in neurological surgery at Johns Hopkins Hospital.

In 1918, Dandy introduced the technique of ventriculography (replacing fluid with air in the ventricles to allow x-ray visualization) as a means of improving diagnosis and subsequently injected air into the spinal canal (pneumoencephalography).[16] The combination of the two modalities expanded the capability for diagnosis of a wide variety of intracranial tumors.

Dandy also advanced surgical techniques in neurosurgery. In 1938, he was the first to selectively obliterate a cerebral aneurysm while preserving flow through the main artery that supplies the area.[17] He applied a simple metal clip that had been introduced by Harvey Cushing in 1911. Dandy also defined the cause of hydrocephalus (the accumulation of an excessive amount of cerebrospinal fluid in the ventricles of the brain).[18] He went on to devise the successful operation of draining the third ventricle of the brain.[19]

Another figure in neurosurgery was Leo M. Davidoff of New York City, who published *The Normal Encephalogram* (1937) and *The Abnormal Encephalogram* (1950), which established him as the father of neuroradiology in North America. In 1955, with the aid of Eugene Spitz, a machine shop technician, and John Holter, whose infant required treatment for hydrocephalus, Davidoff developed a one-way silicon valve that expedited the drainage of the excessive fluid.[20] An engineering accomplishment that was stimulated by personal concern was thus added to the therapeutic armamentarium.

A more common clinical concern of neurosurgery is the rupture of an intervertebral disk (the cartilaginous material between the vertebrae of the spine). In 1911, far in advance of his time, Joel E. Goldthwaite of Boston was the first to postulate that sciatic pain could be caused by dislocation of a lumbar disk in the vertebral canal.[21] The first reported successful treatment is credited to both Boston neurosurgeon William J. Mixter and orthopaedic surgeon Joseph S. Barr, who conjointly established the degenerative origin of the lesion and its relationship to sciatic nerve pain.[22]

PLASTIC AND RECONSTRUCTIVE SURGERY

Meaningful contributions were made in plastic and reconstructive surgery before the specialty was defined as a distinct entity. In 1881, Edward Talbot Ely of Manhattan Eye, Ear, and Throat Hospital, described in the literature for the first time an operation for the correction of prominent ears.[23] Two decades later, William H. Luckett of Lutheran Hospital in New York City introduced a new concept in the treatment of protruding ears, one that has formed the basis for all subsequent approaches.[24] In 1887, Thomas L. Gilmer, at the time a physician-dentist working at the College of Medicine in Quincy, Illinois, and later dean at the Northwestern University Dental School, reported for the first time fixation of a fractured mandible (lower jaw) by wiring the lower teeth to the upper teeth to prevent movement.[25]

Vilray Papin Blair of Washington University in St. Louis is known as the Father of American Plastic Surgery. In 1909, he published a revolutionary technique for the correction of an underdeveloped lower jaw with limited excursion.[26] He produced three classic volumes in the field of plastic surgery: *Surgery and Diseases of the Mouth and Jaws* (1912), *Essentials of Oral Surgery* (1923), and *Cancer of the Face and Mouth* (1941). Blair established the first plastic surgery service in the United States and perhaps in the world. Among his trainees was Earl C. Padgett, who subsequently headed the plastic surgery department at the University of Kansas Medical School and whose name is associated with the "drum" dermatome devised for removing large sheets of skin to be used in grafting.

Pediatric Surgery

In pediatric surgery, William E. Ladd of Boston Children's Hospital introduced a procedure to correct malrotation of the intestines (in which the intestine is twisted on itself and consequently obstructed).[27] Both William E. Ladd and N. Logan Leven of St. Paul, Minnesota, are credited with the first successful repair of a tracheoesophageal fistula (a track between the trachea, or windpipe, and the esophagus, or gullet, usually associated with absence of part of the esophagus) by ligating the fistula, placing a tube for feeding into the stomach, and repairing the esophagus at a later date.[28] Cameron Haight in Ann Arbor, Michigan, performed the first successful primary (at an initial operation) reestablishment of continuity for esophageal atresia (absence of part of the esophagus).[29] Dr. Orvar Swenson of Chicago gained eponymic fame for devising an operation to treat Hirschprung's disease, characterized by the absence of ganglia, usually in the lower portion of the colon (large intestine).[30]

In the early 1980s, Michael Harrison of the University of California, San Francisco, initiated a new revolutionary field in pediatric surgery. Intrauterine operations on the fetus offered therapeutic options for several congenital anomalies. The advent of minimal access surgical techniques in 1989 offered the opportunity to reduce both maternal morbidity and the risk of inducing premature labor. The minimal access techniques have been referred to as fetal endoscopy, or by the abbreviation FETENDO.

Currently, the lesions that have been successfully repaired in the fetus include obstruction of the outflow of the urinary bladder, congenital diaphragmatic hernia, congenital cystic adenomatoid malformation (a cystic tumor of the lung that can compromise respiration), large saccrococcygeal teratomas (tumors of embryonic germ layers in the region of the coccyx and sacrum), and myelomeningocele (a hernia of the spinal cord and its coverings through the posterior vertebral column).[31] When monozygotic twins share a single placenta, they also share vascular connections that increase mortality and morbidity. Fetoscopic techniques have been applied to ablate the vascular connections and prevent adverse consequences. Advances in intrauterine surgery await additional technical refinement to expand their applicability.

The advances in the surgical specialties that have been discussed in this chapter, when added to the modernization of vascular surgery, the establishment of cardiothoracic surgery, and the initiation of all aspects of organ transplantation, allow for the conclusion that there is no aspect of modern surgery that has not been impacted by American ingenuity and innovation. If we then invoke the earlier significant contributions that took place during the nineteenth century, the total effect is analogous to a broad landscape replete with elegant details.

CHAPTER 13:

ENABLING EXPANSION

The constancy of the internal environment is the condition of free and independent existence.

—Claude Bernard
Leçons sur les phénomènes de la vie communs aux animaux et aux végétaux (1878)

The significant contributions of American surgeons presented in this book—with the exception of William Beaumont's clinical experimentation that defined gastric digestion and the introduction of surgical anesthesia—have focused on technical feats that have kept with the general image of the surgeon as a brilliant craftsman. This aura that surrounds the surgeon is, to a large extent, a product of the patient's psyche. This is because during most operations patients are anesthetized and disconnected from any personal involvement in the situation. As such, they are reliant solely on the surgeon to separate them from their disease or to repair an injury. The patient's life is literally in the surgeon's hands and the surgeon's reputation is based on his or her facility with the instruments he or she uses to heal the patient during operative procedures.

The praiseworthy surgeons identified in the previous chapters are indeed notable because of the technical accomplishments achieved by their gifted hands. These surgeons, however, are not mere craftsman and should be commended as well for their just as gifted minds.

For instance, as the complexity of surgical procedures has increased, the surgeon's appreciation of the physiologic implications of putting the patient "under the knife" has also grown. For all operations, the time period of the procedure and the time immediately surrounding the event is known as the perioperative period and is flanked by preoperative and postoperative periods. As the spectrum of surgical procedures has increased in diversity and complexity, the surgeon has had to increase attention to each of these three periods of care. The ability of patients to withstand an operation, regardless of its complexity, has also increased. Age is now rarely a limiting factor and impaired function can usually be rectified to the extent that almost any patient can tolerate almost any operation. Whatever the age or state of a patient may be, he or she still requires the surgeon to make precise physiologic adjustments in order to reduce the risks of a complex operation.

One example of what a surgeon has to adjust because of the increase in the length and complexity of an operation is a patient's bodily fluids. Extensive removal of tissue and organs, intricate and prolonged reparative and reconstructive procedures, operations on the heart and the major blood vessels, and the transplantation of organs are all associated with the potential need to replace blood loss. These changes may also involve the patient's plasma volume, extracellular fluid, and electrolytes. The surgeon must account for all of these in order to maintain equilibrium within the internal environment of the patient's body.

In addition to bodily fluids, physiologic changes in cardiac, vascular, respiratory, hepatic, and renal function often occur during the course of a complex procedure. These physiological alterations may continue or even amplify during the patient's period of recovery. The replacement of blood or its components, the maintenance of appropriate body fluid volume, electrolyte levels, and the provision of adequate nutritional essentials have become requisite accompaniments to complex operations. Thus, surgeons must prepare for the impact that all procedures and their concomitant effects have on a body's homeostasis.

Every one of these issues is a component of the metabolic alteration that the patient undergoes during an operation. These changes and complications, which often are increased during the postoperative period, may require the management of an intensive care unit to expedite recovery. As is implicit in the name, activities in that location mandate a surgeon and the team's in-depth appreciation of physiologic changes and therapeutic interventions.

Over the course of time, American surgery and medicine has contributed significantly to the appreciation and management of the changes and problems consequent to surgical procedures. Participants in this arena have included many American surgeons. It is the innovations of these surgical scientists that have played a critical role in enabling the ensuing technical virtuosity of the gifted hands explored previously in this book. Harvey Cushing was prescient when he wrote: "I would like to see the day when somebody would be appointed surgeon somewhere who had no hands, for the operative part is the least part of the work."[1]

We will explore several of the areas outside the realm of surgical technique to which American surgeons have made significant contributions and thereby allowed for the expansion of surgery.

Blood

Maintenance of the volume and the components of blood in surgical patients throughout their care is mandatory. The statement in Deuteronomy 11:23, "The blood is the life," indicates the ancients' appreciation of this vital suspension. The beginning of transfusion therapy resulted from a publication by William Harvey in 1628. He explained that blood circulated throughout the body in a closed system in which the heart acted as a pump and propelled oxygenated red blood cells through arteries peripherally to all tissues and organs. From these, the blood returned via the veins to the heart.

In 1667, the first recorded transfusion took place in France, when physician Jean-Baptiste Denis infused blood from a sheep into a fifteen-year-old who had been bled many times as treatment for fever—the patient improved. Almost simultaneously, Richard Lower, an Oxford physician, demonstrated to the Royal Society in London a transfusion from a sheep's artery to a human. Back in France, Denis repeated with a second success but followed with two deaths subsequent to the transfusion of animal blood. These deaths led the Paris Society of Physicians to forbid the procedure. In 1678, the Royal Society in England followed suit.

After a hiatus of one hundred fifty years, James Blundell, a London obstetrician, reinstituted transfusion experiments and concluded that only human blood should be employed for humans. He used venous blood administered by syringes and tubes and achieved success in five of ten patients treated for blood loss. As noted earlier, William Stewart Halsted in 1881 transfused his sister, who was hemorrhaging after delivery of her first child, with his own blood that was administered via a syringe. In all cases, these patients were most fortunate that there was no major incompatibility with the donor blood. Two years later, Halsted reported the first successful case of reinfusion of an individual's own blood.

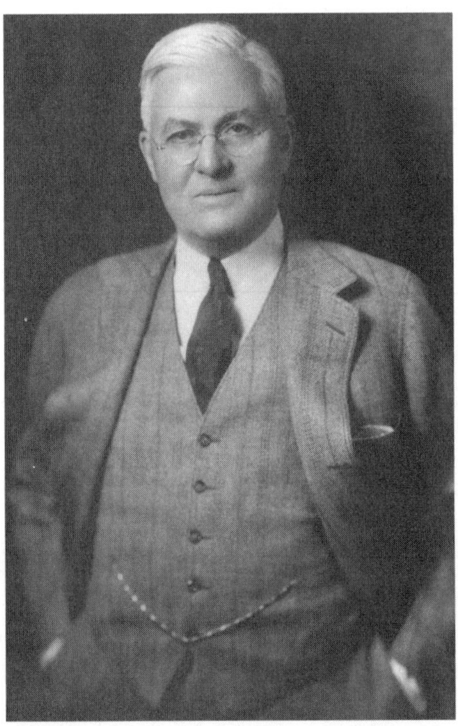

Figure 42: George W. Crile. Courtesy of the Cleveland Clinic.

In 1901, while working in the University of Vienna Department of Pathological Anatomy, Karl Landsteiner discovered the blood groups, which he called A, B, and C (later A, B, and O). Although Landsteiner indicated that the clumping of red cells by incompatible serum might explain previously noted adverse reactions to transfusions, the discovery failed to have an impact on transfusion therapy for over a decade. In 1930, Landsteiner received the Nobel Prize for Physiology or Medicine for his contribution. A decade later, he and Alexander S. Wiener identified the rhesus (Rh) factor and the anti-Rh antibody.[2]

In 1908, the distinguished surgeon and founder of the Cleveland Clinic, George W. Crile (fig. 42), published an extraordinary book of 560 pages detailing his laboratory and clinical experiences.[3] He reported sixty-one direct transfusions in fifty-five patients using a metal tube through which arterial blood from donors passed into the recipients' veins. Before most of the medical profession accepted and applied the importance of Karl Landsteiner's previous findings related to blood typing, Crile performed hemolysis testing between donor and recipient blood to determine compatibility prior to proceeding with a transfusion.

Most patients transfused were those with septic, trauma-associated, or hemorrhagic shock. Crile was prescient in his analysis that "transfusion may easily succeed when saline infusions completely fail."[4] He concluded: "In uncomplicated hemorrhage, when treated *before the central nervous system has become irreparably damaged by anemia*, transfusion is a specific remedy."[5]

After an appreciation of the importance of the blood groups was widely

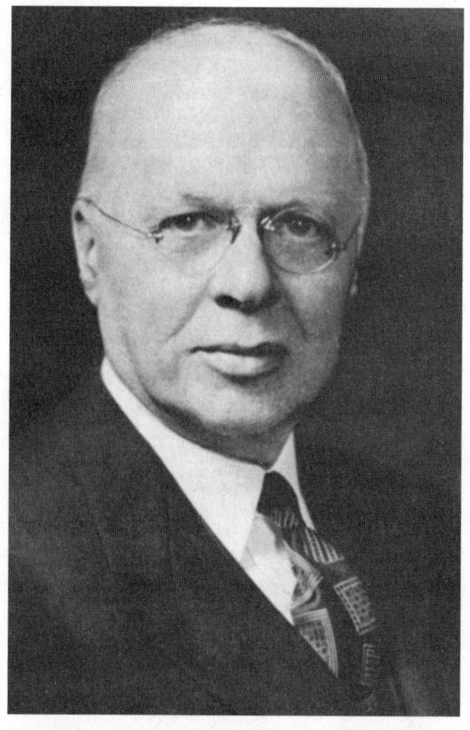

Figure 43: Richard Lewisohn. Courtesy of the Mount Sinai Archives.

accepted, attention was directed at methods for preserving blood so that it was conveniently available to replace the acute blood loss occurring in association with trauma or during surgical operations. The initial resolution of this requirement is credited to Richard Lewisohn (fig. 43), a native of Germany, who performed his work at Mount Sinai Hospital in New York City. In 1915, Lewisohn introduced the sodium citrate method of blood preservation.[6] He demonstrated that a massive transfusion of 2,500 mL of citrated blood could be given safely in a short period. The citation for the Karl Landsteiner Award, which he received in 1955, reads: "For distinguished contribution to the field of blood-banking in discovering the use of sodium citrate as an anticoagulant which made possible the safe and effective storage of blood and the subsequent development of blood banks. A milestone in the history of medical science which has saved countless lives both in war and in peace and which has made possible further advances in medical and surgical treatment of disease."

On a side note, Lewisohn is also credited with having persuaded A. A. Berg of Mount Sinai Hospital to perform the first removal of a part of the stomach as treatment for peptic ulcer in the United States. Lewisohn noted that, after partial removal, the contents of the stomach lost their acidity. He also suggested infection as a possible cause of peptic ulcer in 1925, sixty years before the role of *Helicobacter pylori* bacteria was defined.[7]

The next phase of blood banking addressed the issue of long-term storage by the freezing of red cells. Frozen red cells have the advantage of increased length of storage. The process also allows for the accumulation of large quantities of O Rh-negative red blood cells (or universal donor) devoid of plasma and leukocytes. The use of frozen blood was first reported in 1965 by Charles Huggins, a surgeon at Massachusetts General Hospital and the son of the Nobel laureate of the same name. [8]

FLUID AND ELECTROLYTES

When the hemoglobin containing red blood cells are removed from the blood, the plasma that courses through the body's vascular channels has a drab straw color. The fluid in the extracellular and intracellular spaces is colorless. The charged elements that make up the electrolytes within these body fluids are invisible. But physiologically, fluids and electrolytes are colorful and dynamic elements that are paramount to the care of the surgical patient. Changes in fluid volume and electrolyte composition can occur in response to trauma, overwhelming infection, or surgical operations. Attention to the details of managing deficits, excesses, or inappropriate proportions continues throughout the preoperative, intraoperative, and postoperative periods.

The origin of the current appreciation of postoperative fluid therapy is hard to pinpoint. In 1907, John H. Gibbon, professor of surgery at Jefferson Medical College and father of the developer of the heart-lung machine, indicated that fluid therapy was becoming an integral component of postoperative care.[9] In 1923, Wilder Penfield and David Teplitsky administered intermittent infusions of 800 to 1,500 mL of normal saline solution, or 5 percent glucose in water, postoperatively during a two- to four-hour period, monitoring venous pressure during the occasion.[10]

A year later, Rudolph Matas (see chapter 9) pointed out the shortcomings of proctoclysis (administration of fluid per rectum) and hypodermoclysis (subcutaneous fluid administration), which were prevalent at the time. He prescribed instead the continuous administration of 4,000 to 5,000 mL per twenty-four hours of preferably a 5 percent glucose solution through a glass tube into an arm vein.[11]

The genesis of modern fluid therapy in surgical patients, however, is often traced to James L. Gamble, a pediatrician at Massachusetts General Hospital. His initial stimulus stemmed from an implication of the importance of fluid and electrolytes in the pathophysiology of pyloric obstruction (obstruction of the outlet of the stomach in the newborn) and infantile diarrhea. Fluid and electrolyte deficits were the direct causes of the lethality associated with these two disorders. Gamble's studies led to his classic tome, *Chemical Anatomy, Physiology and Pathology of Extracellular Fluid* (1947).[12]

Early in the evolution of the fluid therapy that was associated with surgical operations, a distinct preference for 5 percent glucose solution prevailed, while there was an opposition to the use of saline solutions. Frederick Coller, the chair of surgery at the University of Michigan, and his associate Walter Maddock were the first to focus on the insensible loss (loss of fluid and electrolytes through the lungs and skin and not readily measurable) during the operative and postoperative periods and emphasized the need for replacement. In time, salt solutions were appropriately used in surgical patients. Up to the mid-twentieth century, Coller's formula for fluid and electrolyte therapy in the postoperative period, with an emphasis on salt restriction, dominated. Carl Moyer brought attention to the internal distribution of fluid and electrolytes and the fact that the changes, in the absence of any external losses, could impair renal function.[13]

In a classic review, Henry T. Randall, chair of surgery at Memorial Hospital in New York and, subsequently, chair of surgery at Brown University Medical School, defined the mid-twentieth-century status of fluid and electrolyte therapy and described the functional divisions of bodily fluid. [14] His measurements of total-body water, the size of the extracellular and intracellular fluid spaces, and the concentration of electrolytes were based on dilutional studies initiated by Francis D. Moore. After presenting the baseline requirements and an analysis of the external losses and fluid shifts that accompany a prolonged operation and extend into the postoperative period, the appropriate use of diverse electrolytes and fluids was detailed. He emphasized the need to correct for loss of potassium.

Shortly thereafter, G. Tom Shires (fig. 44), who is distinguished for serving as chair of four surgical departments (University of Texas Southwestern Medial School, University of Washington, Cornell University, and Texas Tech University) and president of the American College of Surgeons and American Surgical Association, demonstrated something of paramount significance. He asserted if appropriate amounts of blood, fluid, and electrolytes were administered during an operation or in the treatment of shock associated with trauma and extracellular fluid volume, homeostasis could be maintained and postoperative renal failure could be avoided.[15] He and his associates rejuvenated the use of saline solutions in which the electrolytes

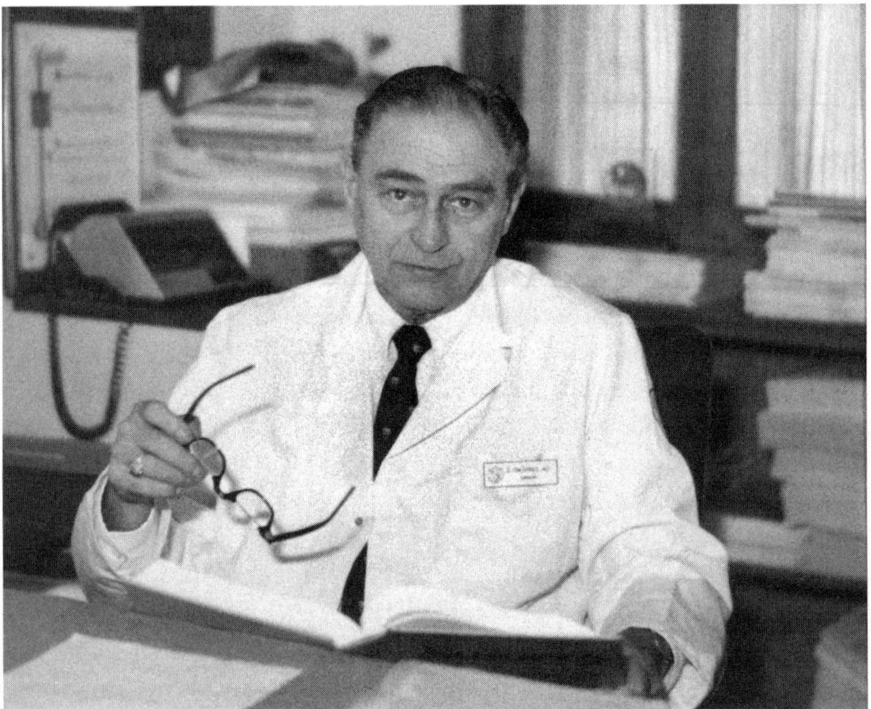

Figure 44: G. Tom Shires. Courtesy of Stephen E. Ettinghausen.

were balanced. The era of severe restriction of fluid and salt in the postoperative period that dominated the earlier fifties thus came to an end.

BURNS

Mastering fluid and electrolyte therapy was also of critical importance in the management of burns. The immediate survival of patients with burns covering a large surface area is, to the greatest extent, dependent on appropriate intravenous infusions. The seminal extensive assessment of "burn shock" associated with fluid and electrolyte shifts is attributed to Franklin H. Underhill, a professor of pharmacology and toxicology at Yale University. His findings stemmed from studies of twenty patients who were victims of a fire in the Rialto Theater in New Haven, Connecticut, in 1921.

Underhill demonstrated that the shock associated with major burns was the result of fluid and electrolyte translocations from the circulation to the extravascular spaces around the burn. He advised that large quantities of saline solutions should be administered intravenously. His work shifted the focus of the treatment of burned patients from the then contemporary theory that toxins caused the shock to fluid resuscitation.[16]

Twenty-one years after the New Haven fire, another fire catalyzed another significant American contribution to the fluid therapy of burns. The Cocoanut Grove fire, which took place at a nightclub in Boston on Novemeber 28, 1942, remains the deadliest night club fire in the history of the United States, killing 492 people and injuring hundreds more. The entire June 1943 issue of the *Annals of Surgery* addressed the diverse aspects of care for the burn victims at Massachusetts General Hospital. Using sophisticated measurements of the body's fluid spaces and the external wound losses of the patients treated there, Oliver Cope and Francis D. Moore developed the first formula for fluid therapy based on body surface area for patients with a burn of 15 percent or more of the body surface.[17]

In 1952, Everett I. Evans of Richmond, Virginia, devised the first surface area–weight formula for computing fluid replacement in burn patients.[18] His regimen was based upon replacement that used normal saline and albumin (colloid), along with 5 percent dextrose in water to cover insensible losses from the skin and lungs. Surgeons at Brooke Army Medical Center in San Antonio, Texas, modified the Evans formula by substituting lactated Ringer's solution for normal saline and decreasing the amount of albumin given; this became the standard for years.[19] The Brooke formula shares popularity with the Parkland formula proposed by Charles Baxter and G. Tom Shires of the University of Texas Southwestern Medical School in Dallas.[20]

The contributions of American surgeons to the care of the burn wounds have been significant. The evolution of early care to prevent bacterial contamination by the applications, initially, of silver nitrate, later mafenide acetate (Sulfamylon), and subsequently silver sulfadiazine cream all emanated from American surgeons. The first report of a series of cases treated by early excision of the burned area followed by immediate grafting is credited to Oliver Cope and associates.[21] The principle employed initially by James Tanner and his associates in constructing the mesh skin graft to cover large denuded areas remains the standard approach.[22] The most recent American input has been John Burke's development of artificial dermis,

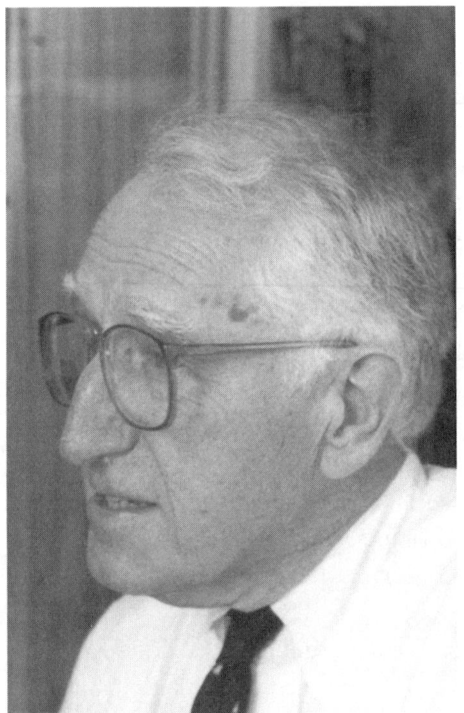

Figure 45: Francis D. Moore. Courtesy of Francis D. Moore Jr.

which is marketed as Integra, to cover the denuded surface after excision of the burned tissue.[23] The artificial dermis has been refined to serve as a matrix for engrafting the patient's own cultured skin cells, creating the first bilaminate skin substitute.[24]

METABOLIC CARE OF THE SURGICAL PATIENT

Most would agree that Francis D. Moore (fig. 45) was the most recognizable and influential surgical physiologist of the twentieth century. During his residency at Massachusetts General Hospital, under the direction of Oliver Cope, he was an integral participant in the management and study of the victims of the Cocoanut Grove fire. Five years after completing his residency, Moore was appointed surgeon-in-chief at Peter Bent Brigham Hospital and the fourth Moseley Professor of Surgery at Harvard Medical School, following in the footsteps of J. Collins Warren, Harvey Cushing, and Elliot C. Cutler.

Without knowing that George von Hevesy at Manchester Physics Laboratories in England had previously published on the measurement of body water using isotopic hydrogen, Moore initiated his own investigations into the matter. He employed a variety of radioactive and nonradioactive isotopes (a form of an element with the same or closely related properties and the same atomic number but different atomic weights), injected them into the subject, and, by determining the extent of dilution, measured the body's component fluid mass and the distribution of electrolytes. This provided more precise data on which replacement therapy could be based.

In 1959, Moore's *Metabolic Care of the Surgical Patient* was published.[25] *Time* referred to it as a six-pound omnibus of 1,011 pages that is essential for modern surgeons. The author's own words spell out the scope of what is probably the largest single-authored surgical text of modern times: "The range of disorders included here covers most of the metabolic situations encountered on a general surgical service plus some of those seen in urology, orthopaedics, and neurosurgery. We have allocated 'fluid balance' to its place as one of several important categories of metabolic management in surgery. Problems of blood volume, visceral disease, nutrition, and severe injury have equal importance in this book as they do on a surgical ward."

The broad scope of the work encompasses many issues, including a consideration of body composition, metabolism, and endocrinology of the resting normal patient. The book also defines convalescence in the healthy patient subjected to soft-tissue trauma of moderate severity, while also presenting variations and abnormalities of convalescent metabolism, including those occurring in the very old and the very young. It focuses also on surgical endocrinology and metabolism and considers metabolic activation after injury.

Nutritional Support

Toward the end of the 1970s, a depiction of the surgical scene would present a broad and diverse panorama that was the result of extraordinary technical advances, as well as an appreciation of the importance of maintaining homeostasis, including blood, extravascular fluid, and electrolyte levels. A missing ingredient required for the expansion of the surgical canvas, however, was nutritional support. Poorly nourished patients, who were unable to correct the deficiencies through oral or tube feeding into the intestine, required nutritional support in order to tolerate extensive surgical procedures. The same support was considered essential in anticipation of the potential morbidities and prolonged care of patients undergoing complex procedures.

In a landmark paper published in 1968, Stanley Dudrick and associates observed six puppies that were fed entirely intravenously for 72 to 256 days and compared them to their orally fed littermates.[26] The intravenously fed puppies outstripped their controls in weight and equaled them in development. Intravenous alimentation was then extended to human patients with success. The essence of the contribution was the threading of the catheter from the external jugular vein in the neck into the superior vena cava (the vein that drains all of the upper body and limbs into the heart), which had sufficient dimensions and flow to permit the infusion of a hypertonic, high-caloric fluid without clotting the vessel. The birth of total parenteral nutrition (TPN) was critical in the expansion of surgery.

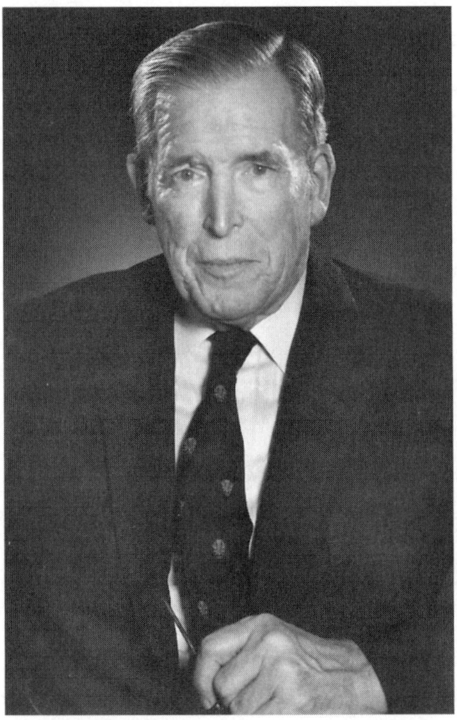

Figure 46: Jonathan E. Rhoads. Courtesy of Clyde F. Barker.

This work was conducted under the direction of Jonathan E. Rhoads (fig. 46), professor and chair of surgery at the University of Pennsylvania and one of the giants of American surgery. Not only was he honored with the presidency of many surgical societies, including the American Surgical Association and the American College of Surgeons, plus innumerable distinguished awards, but he was also the second and only other American surgeon (W. W. Keen was the first, from 1908–1918) to serve as president of the American Philosophical Society (1976–1984), the nation's oldest scholarly organization.

EXTRACORPOREAL MEMBRANE OXYGENATION (ECMO)

ECMO, which is generally attributed to Robert H. Bartlett, professor of surgery at the University of Michigan, offers the most successful method of compensating for the respiratory failure associated with congenital diaphragmatic hernia in a newborn until the newborn can tolerate operative correction. The applicability of this technique transcends the surgical domain and has broad application for other causes of impaired respiration.

Bartlett's work on ECMO began in 1965 at Peter Bent Brigham Hospital with attempts to improve the efficiency of artificial membrane oxygenators. Clinical trials with ECMO were initiated by Bartlett and his surgical colleague Alan Gazzaniga of the University at California, Irvine, in 1972. The first clinical cases in which ECMO was used for cardiopulmonary support in infancy were reported in 1976. After Bartlett moved to the University of Michigan in 1980, there was a rapid increase in the number and diversity of situations for which infants were managed by this modality. This method afforded a survival rate of 90 percent for cases of neonatal respiratory failure, frequently a consequence of meconium (the first fecal material consisting of amniotic fluid, mucus, bile, and sloughed intestinal cells) aspiration, and a 70 percent survival rate for patients treated because of the impaired development of the lung associated with diaphragmatic hernia.[27]

ANTI-ANGIOGENESIS

The term "anti-angiogenesis" literally means "against the formation of blood vessels." Most would agree that the premier and most consummate surgical researcher into this matter since its inception in the second half of the twentieth century was Judah Folkman (fig. 47), whose death, sadly, occurred precisely during the preparation of this section. As a student at Harvard Medical School, Folkman developed the first atrioventricular implantable pacemaker for the heart. Before completing his surgical residency, he reported the use of implantable silicone-rubber polymers for the sustained release of drugs. The research findings served as the basis for controlled release drug therapy and also for

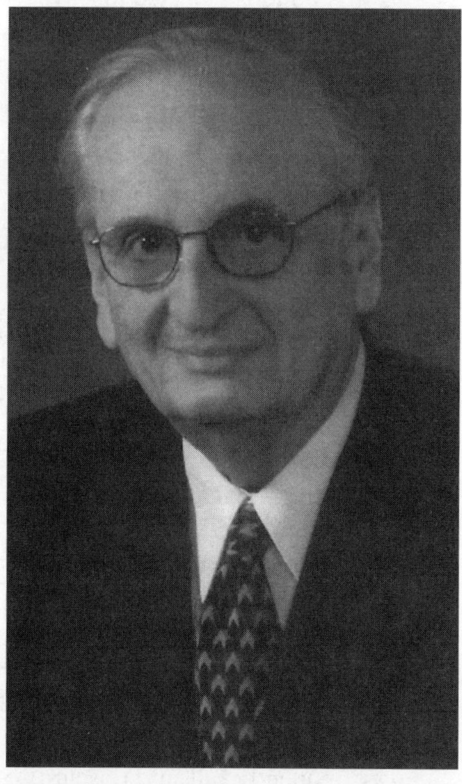

Figure 47: Judah Folkman. Courtesy of Arthur J. Moss and the Judah Folkman family.

Norplant, the five-year implantable contraceptive. Folkman completed his residency at Massachusetts General Hospital in 1965 and, two years later, he was appointed surgeon-in-chief at Boston Children's Hospital, a position he held for fourteen years.

In 1971, Folkman's initial paper on angiogenesis was published.[28] In it he wrote: "Tumor cells appear to stimulate endothelial-cell proliferation, and endothelial cells may have an indirect effect over the rate of tumor growth." He reported the isolation of a tumor-angiogenesis factor (TAF) from human and animal tumors. In the same paper, Folkman proposed the term "anti-angiogenesis" to mean prevention of new vessel sprouts from penetrating into early tumor implants. He concluded with characteristic humility: "Anti-angiogenesis may provide a form of cancer therapy worthy of serious exploration."

In 1981, Folkman elected to leave the operating theater for the laboratory and became director of the vascular biology program at Boston Children's Hospital and professor of cell biology at Harvard Medical School. The laboratory that he has directed for the past three decades has been extraordinarily productive. Investigators in the laboratory purified the first angiogenic protein from a tumor, identified the first angiogenesis inhibitor, purified the first angiogenic molecule, and initiated clinical trials in which anti-angiogenic agents were used to control tumor growth.

As indicated in Folkman's presidential address to the American Association of Pediatric Surgeons in May 2006, at least eight anti-angiogenic agents are approved for cancer therapy in the United States and some are currently used in thirty other countries.[29] Exciting results have also been reported for the use of anti-VEGF antibody, an anti-angiogenic drug, as treatment for so-called wet, age-related macular degeneration, which is characterized by formation of new retinal blood vessels.

—ꟺ—

The impact of the above-mentioned surgeons on the success of surgical procedures is enormous but lacks the visibility of the more illustrious technical feats explored earlier in this book. As a consequence, the names of surgical scientists frequently fall into obscurity, an obscurity that is unjustified since there would have been no surgical progress without their accomplishments.

—ꟺ—

In discussing the past contributions of American surgeons who had a significant impact on medicine, I have attempted to be inclusive, but, of course, there remains an element of personal selectivity. A window into the assessment of others in reference to the more recent contributions is appropriate. Following World War II, the Albert Lasker Research Award for Basic and Clinical Research and Public Service was established and has been awarded annually. Informally, the award has come to be known as the "American Nobel Prize for Physiology or Medicine." Included on the list of former winners are several surgeons whose names have appeared previously in this narrative.

The surgical recipients of the Lasker Award, in chronological order, are as follows: in 1954, Alfred Blalock and Robert E. Gross with Helen B. Taussig for their advances in cardiovascular disease; in 1955, C. Walton Lillehei and Richard L. Varco for advances in cardiovascular surgery; in 1963, Michael E. DeBakey for advances in cardiovascular surgery and Charles B. Huggins for hormonally based surgical treatment of advanced prostatic and breast cancer treatment; in 1967, John H. Gibbon Jr. for creating the heart-lung machine; in 1984, Henry J. Heimlich for developing the maneuver that prevents death from choking; in 1985, Bernard Fisher for shaping the modern treatment of breast cancer; in 2000, Harold P. Freeman for enlightening scientists and the public about the relationship between race, poverty, and cancer; and in 2007, Albert Starr (shared with Alain Carpentier) for creating prosthetic heart valves.

The United States Postal Service has provided another vehicle for the recognition of some American surgeons by the issuance of commemorative stamps. A total of seven surgeons are represented on six such stamps. The selection is totally unpredictable and, doubtlessly, politically biased. The first of the surgeon stamps depicted Crawford Long on a 2-cent stamp in 1940. In 1949, Ephraim McDowell's portrait appeared on a 4-cent stamp. This was followed in 1964 by the profiles of the Mayo Brothers, William J. and Charles H., on a 5-cent stamp. In 1981, Charles Drew, the African American surgeon who chaired the department of surgery at Howard University, was pictured on a 35-cent stamp. A year later, Mary Walker, who had received the Medal of Honor for her activities as a medical officer with the Union Army, was honored by a 20-cent stamp. Finally, Harvey Cushing's portrait appeared in 1990 on a 45-cent stamp.

One of the popularly accepted criteria of notability or significance is appearance on the cover of *Time* magazine. The September 16, 1935, issue featured the first surgical portrait—that of Alexis Carrel. After a hiatus of over twenty years, Charles P. Bailey appeared on the cover of the March 25, 1957, issue. Francis D. Moore was depicted on the May 3, 1963, cover. Subsequently, Michael E. DeBakey, appeared on the May 25, 1965, cover, and William DeVries, on December 10, 1984, completed the roster, the former for his many contributions to vascular surgery and the latter for the insertion of an artificial heart.

Our journey through the past of American surgery has come to an end. The seminal and significant contributions that have taken place in the two hundred years between Ephraim McDowell's operation on Jane Todd Crawford and today have been most impressive and often groundbreaking. The last two centuries have provided surgical innovations that have comforted patients, extended their lives, and improved the quality of their lives. The ingenuity of American surgeons and the intellectual fertility of American soil have proved to be a dynamic and praiseworthy combination that holds promise for the future.

ON THE HORIZON

The glory of medicine is that it is constantly moving forward, that there is always more to learn.

—William J. Mayo
National Education Association: Addresses and Proceedings (1928)

As a member of the group of older surgeons who has witnessed the extraordinary panoply of discoveries, innovations, and refinements that have evolved during our surgical lives, I can only conclude that future contributions will outstrip our wildest estimates. During our time, the number of individuals capable of introducing radical departures or meaningful changes in concepts and techniques has greatly multiplied. Future generations of surgeons will have an ever-increasing technical and scientific platform from which to innovate. Furthermore, the psychologic profile of the young surgeon is that of a less constrained, less orthodox, and more adventuresome individual. Tradition has been replaced by trials. More adventuresome surgeons, with the aid of more advanced technologies, will create change at an accelerated pace.

The next fifty years certainly will witness many barely imaginable additions and changes in surgery. Other advances that surely will become standard are already in embryonic stages. Within all the surgical specialties, the safety of the more complex and challenging operative interventions will increase. For instance, the production and applicability of chemical compounds with the physiologic attributes of red blood cells should come to pass. Pharmacologically produced hemoglobin, which has been the object of research over the past three decades, will provide a substrate that can transport oxygen for cellular activity and remove the carbon dioxide in cases of severe blood loss. Similarly, artificial cells or combinations of organic chemicals may replicate many of the functions of platelets and white blood cells, such as maintaining normal blood clotting and defense against infection, respectively.

The critical postoperative period also will change. Detection of changes will be improved by modifications in the monitoring of patients, which will be introduced in more-sophisticated intensive care units. Wireless connections and nanotechnology will reduce the lag time between critical changes in patients on those units and the recognition of those changes by the responsible medical personnel. Small chips, which are worn by or implanted in patients, might provide immediate detection and transmission of physiologic alterations to centralized and satellite stations. These advances should be synergistic with the physician's ability to care for critically ill patients.

The same nanotechnology and implanted chips will also increase the safety of trauma care. An awareness by the trauma team of altered organ function or medications in injured patients, who are unable to communicate because of unresponsiveness, will be expedited. All individuals will have an electronic profile of their past medical history and current medications. Accordingly, treatment could be modified in order to minimize adverse effects. On the opposite end of the spectrum of patient care, the same technology will be used to detect and transmit to a central station pertinent changes in electrophysiologic and biochemical data of patients after discharge from the hospital. Delay of treatment will be avoided.

In the realm of changes in surgical techniques, sutured intestinal anastomosis may become a procedure of the past with the perfection of mechanical coapting devices and the use of more compatible and effective glues and tissue sealants that can be applied laparoscopically or endoscopically. Refinements in equipment and techniques will result in the extension of indications for minimally invasive approaches to removal of all or a part of many organs within the abdomen and chest. Removal of the pancreas and parts of the liver might be routinely performed by the laparoscopic approach. It is already apparent that the minimally invasive endovascular approach will become the standard for most operations on major blood vessels.

Natural orifice translaparoscopic enteric surgery (NOTES), which is a surgery devoid of visible incisions through the skin, is in its infancy and awaits development. Intrauterine surgery, which also awaits complete development, may correct congenital defects or permit genetic manipulation of the fetus to obviate inherited defects in metabolism. After birth, critical metabolic defects might be managed with an artificial pancreas for diabetes or cultured liver cells for hepatic failure. Effective cellular implants of pancreatic islets, liver cells, or stem cells that have the potential to differentiate into islets or liver cells could become routine.

Improvement in vascular techniques and perfusion of whole organs with solutions to maintain viability for prolonged periods of time will permit more liberal application of so-called back-table surgery. This will allow greater facility in a more exposed state, which will then allow an organ to be removed, operated on without blood loss, and then repositioned into its original location.

Transplantation might be facilitated by inducing tolerance preoperatively in order to obviate the need for lifelong immunosuppression. The ultimate resolution of the problem of an insufficient number of donors may be a sequitur of induced tolerance in that compatible grafts from other species will be usable.

Dramatic advances in neurological surgery will be achieved related to spinal cord injury and peripheral nerve regeneration, and, for those with Alzheimer's and Parkinson's disease, intracerebral injections of cells and biochemical manipulations may forestall progression. Improved nerve stimulation, applied through the skin, will control pain more effectively. External electrical stimulation for motor function will be developed. Intractable hypertension might be managed by transmitting neural traffic up the nerves that control blood pressure.

Robotic surgery, which has already become the standard for prostatectomy in younger patients and has seen application in cardiac surgery, will become more widespread. In fact, robotic surgery with its built-in magnification and mechanical precision will spread to all the surgical specialties. A dramatic extension of the robotic technology will be refinements in the capability of performing remote operations by surgeons who are physically distant from the patient. With endovascular techniques, the replacement of heart valves using valvular devices, which are passed to the heart from an artery in the leg, will be more frequently employed.

Today's older surgeons have been a part of what they consider to be the Golden Age of Surgery. The unimaginable has come to pass in an amazingly short period of time. The boundaries of surgery appear limitless. Younger and future surgeons can look forward to an increasing number of even more brilliant advances that will take place in the next fifty years. The result may be an equivalent or even more expansive laudatory designation for the next surgical age.

ENDNOTES

PREFACE

1. Quote taken from Karel B. Absolon, *The Surgeon's Surgeon: Theodor Billroth 1829–1890* (Lawrence, KS: Coronado Press, 1981), p. 186.

CHAPTER 1

1. For description of the Edwin Smith Papyrus see James Henry Breasted, *The Edwin Smith Surgical Papyrus, Published in Facsimile and Hieroglyphics Transliteration with Translation and Commentary* (Chicago: University of Chicago Press, 1930).

2. For quote see Virgil J. Vogel, *American Indian Medicine* (Norman, OK: University of Oklahoma Press, 1970), p. 37.

3. For quote and description see John Lawson, *History of North Carolina* (Richmond, VA: Garrett & Massie, 1937), p. 237, and see Aleš Hrdli ka, *Physiological and Medical Observations among the Indians of Southwestern United States and Northern Mexico* (Washington, DC: Bureau of American Ethnology, 1900), p. 233.

4. Lawson, *History of North Carolina*, pp. 210, 234.

5. Reuben Gold Thwaites, *Early Western Travels, 1748–1846*, vol. 2, *John Long's Journal, 1768–1782* (Cleveland: Arthur H. Clark, 1904).

6. Vogel, *American Indian Medicine*, p. 193.

7. Mark Catesby, *The Natural History of Carolina, Florida, and the Bahama Islands* (London: C. Marsh, 1754), p. xv.

8. Vogel, *American Indian Medicine*, p. 196.

9. For quote and history of Cabeza de Vaca's life see Martin A. Favata and Jóse B. Fernández, *The Account: Álvar Nuñez Cabeza de Vaca's Relación* (Houston: Arte Público Press, 1993).

10. A. Scott Earle, ed., *Surgery in America: From the Colonial Era to the Twentieth Century* (New York: Praeger, 1983), pp. 1–3.

11 Ibid., pp. 4–8.

12. For quote see Leonard F. Peltier, "John Jones: An Extraordinary Surgeon," *Surgery* 59 (1966): 633.

CHAPTER 2

1. A. Scott Earle, ed., *Surgery in America: From the Colonial Era to the Twentieth Century* (New York: Praeger, 1983), p. 69.

2. For quote see John Bell, "Philip Syng Physick" in *American Medical Biography: Lives of Eminent Physicians and Surgeons of the Nineteenth Century*, ed. Samuel D. Gross (Philadelphia: Lindsay and Blakiston, 1861), p. 425.

3. For quote see "Thomas A. Horrocks" in *American National Biography*, vol. 17 (New York: Oxford University Press, 1999), p. 459.

4. August Schachner, *Ephraim McDowell: "Father of Ovariotomy" and Founder of Abdominal Surgery* (Philadelphia and London: J. B. Lippincott, 1921), p. 47.

5. Samuel D. Gross, Memorial Oration in Honor of Ephraim McDowell, Louisville, 1879.

6. Schachner, *Ephraim McDowell*, p. 213.

7 Ibid., p. 290.

8. For quote see Ephraim McDowell, "Three Cases of Extirpation of Diseased Ovaria," *Eclectic Repertory and Analytical Revue* 7 (1817): 242.

9. For Edinburgh report, see John Lizars, "Observations on Extirpation of the Ovaria with Cases," *Edinburgh Medical Journal* 22 (1824).

10. For McDowell's initial publication see ibid., pp. 242–44.

11. For McDowell's second publication, see Ephraim McDowell, "Observations of Diseased Ovaria," *Eclectic Repertory and Analytical Review* 9 (1819): 546–53.

12. For quote see Ezra Michener, *Eclectic Repertory and Analytical Review* 8 (1818): 111.

13. For quote see Thomas Henderson, *Eclectic Repertory and Analytical Review* 8 (1818): 545.

14. For quote see McDowell, "Observations on Diseased Ovaria," p. 548.

15. For quote see James Johnson, "Editorial," *London Medical Chirugical Review* (1825): 83.

16. Ibid.

17. For quote see James Johnson, "Editorial," *London Medical Chirugical Review* (1826): 342.

18. For quote see Schachner, *Ephraim McDowell*, p. 245.

CHAPTER 3

1. For Beaumont's records and bedside note see Jesse S. Myer, *Life and Letters of Dr. William Beaumont* (St. Louis: C. V. Mosby, 1912), pp. 107–108.

2. Ibid.

3. Ibid., p. 115.

4. Joseph Lovell, "A Case of Wounded Stomach by Joseph Lovell, Surgeon General, U.S.A." *Medical Recorder* 8 (1825): 14.

5. Myer, *Life and Letters*, p. 117.

6. Ibid.

7. William Beaumont, "Further Experiments in the Case of Alexis St. Martin, Who Was Wounded in the Stomach by a Load of Duck-Shot, Detailed in the *Recorder* for Jan. 1, 1825," *Medical Recorder* 33 (1826): 94.

8. Myer, *Life and Letters*, p. 147.

9. Ibid., p. 167.

10. Ibid., p. 166.

11. For quote see *New York Evening Post*, September 5, 1833.

12. For quote see Andrew Combe, *Experiments and Observations on the Gastric Juice and the Physiology of Digestion by Wm. Beaumont, of the United States Army*, 1 vol. (Edinburgh: 1838).

13. For quote see Myer, *Life and Letters*, p. 198.

Chapter 4

1. For quote see J. Marion Sims, *The Story of My Life* (New York: Appleton and Company, 1886), p. 135.

2. J. Marion Sims, "Operation for Double Congenital Hair Lip," *American Journal of Dental Science* 5 (1844): 51.

3.For quote see Sims, *The Story of My Life,* p. 226.

4. J. Marion Sims, "The Discovery of Anesthesia," *Virginia Medical Monthly* 4 (1877): 81.

5. For quote see Sims, *The Story of My Life,* p. 245.

6. J. Marion Sims, "Treatment of Vesicovaginal Fistula," *American Journal of Medical Science* 23 (1852): 59.

7. J. Marion Sims, *Clinical Notes on Uterine Surgery, with Special Reference to the Management of the Sterile Condition* (New York: W. Wood, 1866).

8. Irwin H. Kaiser, "Reappraisals of J. Marion Sims," *American Journal of Obstetrics and Gynecology* 132 (1978): 883.

9. *American National Biography*, vol. 20 (New York: Oxford University Press, 1999), p. 25.

10. For quotes see G. J. Barker-Benfield, *The Horrors of the Half-Known Life* (New York: Harper & Row, 1976).

11. For quote see D. E. Alexson, "Women as Victims of Medical Experimentation: J. Marion Sims Surgery on Slave Women 1845–1850," *Sage: A Scholarly Journal on Black Women* 2 (1985).

CHAPTER 5

1. For quote see Frank Kells Boland, *The First Anesthetic: The Story of Crawford Long* (Athens: University of Georgia Press, 1950), p. 2.

2. For quote see Paracelsus, *Paracelsi Opera*, vol. 2 (Geneva: 1658), p. 197.

3. For quote see Humphry Davy, *Researches, Chemical and Philosophical, Chiefly concerning Nitrous Oxide* (London: J. Johnson, 1800), p. 556.

4. H. Hickman, *Letter on Suspended Animation* (Ironbridge: W. Smith, 1824).

5. C. W. Long, "An Account of the First Use of Sulphuric Ether by Inhalation as an Anaesthetic in Surgical Operations," *Southern Medical and Surgical Journal* 5 (1849).

6. J. M. Sims, "Discovery of Anesthesia," *Virginia Medical Monthly* 4 (1877): 81.

7. Hugh H. Young, "Long, the Discoverer of Anesthesia: A Presentation of the Original Documents," *Johns Hopkins Hospital Bulletin* 8 (1897): 174.

8. For quote see John Collins Warren, "Inhalation of Ether Vapor for the Prevention of Pain in Surgical Operations," *Boston Medical and Surgical Journal* 35 (1846): 375.

9. H. J. Bigelow, "Insensibility during Surgical Operations Produced by Inhalation," *Boston Medical and Surgical Journal* 35 (1846): 309.

10. See Warren, "Inhalation of Ether," p. 174.

11. For quote see Barbara M. Duncum, *The Development of Inhalation Anesthesia* (London: Oxford University Press, 1947), p. 562.

12. Robert H. Collyer, "Correspondence," *Lancet* 1 (1847): 265.

13. For quote see S. Weir Mitchell, "The Birth and Death of Pain," in *The Complete Works of S. Weir Mitchell* (New York: Century Company, 1914), p. 416.

14. Ibid.

CHAPTER 6

1. For quote see John Stough Bobbs, "Case of Lithotomy of the Gall-Bladder," *Transactions of the Indiana State Medical Society* 18 (1868): 68.

2. For quote see J. Marion Sims, "Cholecystostomy in Dropsy of the Gall-Bladder," *British Journal of Medicine* 1 (1878): 811.

3. Lawson Tait, "Cholecystotomy for Dropsy of the Gall-Bladder Due to Impaction of Gall-Stone," *Lancet* 2 (1879): 729.

4. G. W. H. Kempner, "Affections of the Gall Bladder Tending to Result in Cutaneous Fistula," *Transactions of the Indiana State Medical Society* 29 (1879): 120.

5. A. W. Brayton, "Dr. John S. Bobbs of Indianapolis, the Father of Cholecystotomy: His Original Paper on Lithotomy of the Gall Bladder," *Indiana State Medical Journal* 24 (1899–1900): 177.

6. For early history of appendicitis and appendectomy see J. Lynwood Harrington, "The Vermiform Appendix: Its Surgical History," *Contemporary Surgery* 39 (1991): 36.

7. A. Groves, *All in a Day's Work: Leaves from a Doctor's Notebook* (Toronto: Macmillan, 1934).

8. W. W. Grant, "The Medical and Surgical History of the Appendix Vermiformis," *Colorado Medicine* 30 (1933): 280.

9. Reginald H. Fitz, "Perforating Inflammation of the Vermiform Appendix with Special Reference to Its Early Diagnosis and Treatment," *American Journal of Medical Science* 92 (1886): 108.

10. C. McBurney, "Experience with Early Operative Interference in Cases of Disease of the Vermiform Appendix," *New York State Medical Journal* 50 (1889): 676.

11. A. J. Ochsner, *Handbook of Appendicitis* (Chicago: G. P. Engelhard, 1906).

12. J. B. Murphy, "Two-Thousand Operations for Appendicitis and Deductions from His Personal Experience," *American Journal of Medical Science* 125 (1904): 187.

13. G. R. Fowler, *A Treatise on Appendicitis* (Philadelphia: J. B. Lippincott, 1894).

Chapter 7

1. For quote see Fielding H. Garrison, *John Shaw Billings: A Memoir* (New York: G. P. Putnam's Sons, 1915), p. 337.

2. Ibid., p. 19.

3. Ibid., p. 27.

4. Ibid., p. 65.

5. Ibid., p. 216.

6. Ibid., p. 182.

7. Ibid., p. 225.

8. W. S. Halsted, "Refusion in the Treatment of Carbonic Oxide Poisoning," *New York Medical Journal* 38 (1883): 625.

9. W. S. Halsted, remarks in discussion of Dr. F. Lange's paper, "The Surgical Significance of Gall-Stones," *Johns Hopkins Hospital Bulletin* 8 (1897): 31.

10. W. S. Halsted, "Radical Cure of Hernia," presented at Johns Hopkins Hospital Medical Society, Baltimore, November 4, 1889, *Johns Hopkins Hospital Bulletin* (1890): 12.

11. For quote see W. S. Halsted, *Surgical Papers*, vol. 1 (Baltimore: Johns Hopkins Press, 1924), p. 306.

12. W. S. Halsted, "The Results of Operations for the Cure of Cancer of the Breast Performed at the Johns Hopkins Hospital from June 1889 to January 1894," *Annals of Surgery* 20 (1894): 497.

CHAPTER 8

1. Harvey W. Cushing, "Hematomyelia from Gunshot Wounds," *American Journal of Medical Science* 145 (1898): 654.

2. Harvey W. Cushing, "Concerning the Poisonous Effect of Pure Sodium Chloride Solutions on the Nerve-Muscle Preparations," *American Journal of Physiology* 6, no. 9 (1901): 77.

3. Harvey W. Cushing, "Instruction in Operative Medicine, with the Description of a Course in the Hunterian Laboratory of Experimental Medicine," *Johns Hopkins Hospital Bulletin* 17 (1908): 124.

4. Harvey W. Cushing, "A Method of Total Extirpation of the Gasserian Ganglion for Trigeminal Neuralgia by a Route through the Temporal Fossa and beneath the Middle Meningeal Artery," *Journal of the American Medical Association* 34 (1900): 1035.

5. Harvey W. Cushing, "The Sensory Distribution of the Fifth Cranial Nerve," *Johns Hopkins Hospital Bulletin* 15 (1904): 213.

6. E. A. Codman, "Report of Results in Nontraumatic Surgery of the Brain and Spinal Cord: Observations on the Actual Results of Cerebral Surgery at the Massachusetts General Hospital," *Boston Medical and Surgical Journal* 153 (1905): 74.

7. Harvey W. Cushing, "The Special Field of Neurological Surgery—Five Years Later," *Johns Hopkins Hospital Bulletin* 21 (1910): 325.

8. Harvey W. Cushing, "The Hypophysis Cerebri: Clinical Aspects of Hyperpituitarism and Hypopituitarism," *Journal of the American Medical Association* 21 (1910): 127–69.

9. Harvey W. Cushing, *The Pituitary Body and Its Disorders* (Philadelphia: J. B. Lippincott, 1912).

10. Harvey W. Cushing, *From a Surgeon's Journal 1915–1918* (Boston: Little, Brown, 1936).

11. Harvey W. Cushing, *Tumors of the Nervus Acusticus and the Syndrome of the Cerebellopontine Angle* (Philadelphia and London: W. B. Saunders, 1917).

12. Percival Bailey and Harvey W. Cushing, *A Classification of the Tumors of the Glioma Group on a Histogenetic Basis with a Correlated Study of Prognosis* (Philadelphia, London, and Montreal: J. B. Lippincott, 1926).

13. Harvey W. Cushing, "Electro-surgery as an Aid to the Removal of Intracranial Tumors: With a Preliminary Note on a New Surgical-Current Generator by W. T. Bovie, PhD, Chicago," *Surgery, Gynecology & Obstetrics* 47 (1928): 751.

14. Harvey W. Cushing, *Intracranial Tumors. Notes upon a Series of Two Thousand Verified Cases with Surgical Mortalities Pertaining Thereto* (Springfield, IL: Charles C. Thomas, 1932).

15. For pituitary basophilism see John F. Fulton, *Harvey Cushing: A Biography* (Springfield, IL: Charles C. Thomas, 1946).

16. Harvey W. Cushing, *Meningiomas* (Springfield, IL: Charles C. Thomas, 1932).

17. Harvey W. Cushing, *A Bio-bibliography of Andreas Vesalius* (New York: Schuman's, 1943).

18. Harvey W. Cushing, *Biography of Sir William Osler* (New York and London: Oxford University Press, 1925).

Chapter 9

1. For early history of vascular surgery see Steven Friedman, *A History of Vascular Surgery*, 2nd ed. (Malden, MA: Blackwell Futura, 2005); Fielding H. Garrison, *An Introduction to the History of Medicine*, 4th ed. (Philadelphia: W. B. Saunders, 1929); Ira M. Rutkow, "Valentine Mott (1785–1865): The Father of American Vascular Surgery," *Surgery* 85 (1979): 441.

2. R. Matas, "Traumatic Aneurysm of the Left Brachial Artery," *Medical News Philadelphia* (1888): 462.

3. R. Matas, "An Operation for the Radical Cure of Aneurysm Based on Arteriorraphy," *Annals of Surgery* 37 (1903): 161.

4. R. Matas, "Personal Experiences in Vascular Surgery," *Annals of Surgery* 112 (1940): 802.

5. Isidore Cohn and Herman B. Deutsch, *Rudolph Matas* (Garden City, NY: Doubleday, 1960).

6. John B. Murphy, "Resection of Arteries and Veins Injured in Continuity-End-to-End Suture-Experimental and Clinical Research," *Medical Recorder* 51 (1897): 73.

7. For quote see the foreword to W. Sterling Edwards, *Alexis Carrel Visionary Surgeon* (Springfield, IL: Charles C. Thomas, 1974).

8. J. Dörfler, "Uber Arterieunaht," *Beitrag Zur Klinischen Chirurgie* 25 (1897): 781.

9. A. Carrel, "Anastomose bout a bout de la Jugulaire et de la Carotide Primitive," *Lyon Médical* 99 (1902): 114.

10. C. A. Hufnagel, "Preserved Arterial Homografts," *Bulletin of the American College of Surgeons* 32 (1947): 231.

11. R. E. Gross, A. Bill, and E. C. Perce II, "Methods for Preservation and Transplantation of Arterial Grafts in Dogs: Report of Transplantation of Preserved Arterial Grafts in 19 Human Cases," *Surgery, Gynecology & Obstetrics* 88 (1949): 689.

12. M. E. DeBakey and F. A. Simeone, "Battle Injuries of the Arteries in World War II," *Annals of Surgery* 123 (1946): 534.

13. E. J. Jahnke Jr. and J. M. Howard, "Primary Repair of Major Arterial Injuries," *Archives of Surgery* 66 (1953): 646.

14. F. C. Spencer and R. V. Grewe, "The Management of Arterial Injuries in Battle Casualties," *Annals of Surgery* 141 (1955): 304.

15. A. B. Voorhees Jr., A. Jaretzki III, and A. H. Blakemore, "The Use of Tubes Constructed from Vinyon 'N' Cloth in Bridging Arterial Defects: A Preliminary Report," *Annals of Surgery* 135 (1952): 332.

16. K. J. Strully, E. S. Hurwitt, and H. W. Blankenberg, "Thromboendarterectomy for Thrombosis of the Internal Carotid in the Neck," *Journal of Neurosurgery* 10 (1953): 474.

17. F. W. Blaisdeell and A. D. Hall, "Axillo-Femoral Artery Bypass for Lower Extremity Ischemia," *Surgery* 54 (1963): 563.

18. N. E. Freeman et al., "Thromboendarterectomy for Hypertension Due to Renal Artery Occlusion," *Journal of the American Medical Association* 156 (1954): 1077.

19. W. F. Barker and J. A. Cannon, "An Evaluation of Endarterectomy," *Archives of Surgery* 66 (1953): 488.

20. R. S. Shaw and R. H. Rutledge, "Superior-Mesenteric-Artery Embolectomy in Treatment of Massive Mesenteric Infarction," *New England Journal of Medicine* 257 (1957): 595.

21. T. J. Fogarty et al., "A Method of Extraction of Arterial Emboli and Thrombi," *Surgery, Gynecology & Obstetrics* 116 (1963): 241.

22. J. H. Jacobson and E. L. Suarez, "Microsurgery in the Anastomosis of Small Vessels," *Surgical Forum* 11 (1968): 243.

23. J. C. Parodi, J. C. Palmaz, and H. D. Barone, "Transfemoral Intraluminal Graft Implantation for Abdominal Aortic Aneurysms," *Annals of Vascular Surgery* 5 (1991): 491.

24. F. C. Spencer, "Plication of the Inferior Cava for Pulmonary Embolism," *Surgery* 6 (1967): 188.

25. L. J. Greenfield et al., "Transvenous Management of Pulmonary Embolic Disease," *Annals of Surgery* 180 (1974): 461.

26. A. O. Whipple, "The Problem of Portal Hypertension in Relation to the Hepatosplenopathies," *Annals of Surgery* 122 (1945): 449.

Chapter 10

1. Rudolph Matas, "On the Management of Acute Traumatic Pneumothorax," *Annals of Surgery* 29 (1899): 409.

2. Rudolph Matas, "Artificial Respiration by Direct Intralaryngeal Intubation with a Modified O'Dwyer Tube and a New Graduated Air-Pump in Its Applications to Medical and Surgical Practice," *Annals of Surgery* 31 (1901): 241.

3. S. J. Meltzer and John Auer, "Continuous Respiration without Respiratory Movements," *Journal of Experimental Medicine* 11 (1909): 622.

4. Franz Torek, "The First Successful Case of Resection of the Thoracic Portion of the Oesophagus for Carcinoma," *Surgery, Gynecology & Obstetrics* 16 (1913): 614.

5. Howard Lilienthal, "Resection of the Lung for Suppurative Infections with a Report Based on 31 Operative Cases in Which Resection Was Done or Intended," *Annals of Surgery* 75 (1922): 257.

6. R. Nissen, "Exstirpation eines ganzen Lungenfleugels," *Zentralblatt fur Chirurgie* 47 (1931): 3003.

7. Evarts A. Graham, "Successful Removal of an Entire Lung for Carcinoma of the Bronchus," *Journal of the American Medical Association* 101 (1933): 1971.

8. Alfred Blalock et al., "The Treatment of Myasthenia Gravis by Removal of the Thymus Gland," *Journal of the American Medical Association* 117 (1941): 1529.

9. H. C. Dalton, "Report of a Case of a Stab-Wound of the Pericardium, Terminating in Recovery after Resection of a Rib and Suture of the Pericardium," *Annals of Surgery* 21 (1895): 147.

10. Daniel Hale Williams, "Stab Wound of the Heart and Pericardium—Suture of the Pericardium—Patient Alive Three Years Afterward," *Medical Record* 51 (1897): 437.

11. Luther L. Hill, "A Report of a Case of Successful Suturing of the Heart, and Table of Thirty-seven Other Cases of Suturing by Different Operators with Various Terminations, and the Conclusions Drawn," *Medical Record* 62 (1902): 846.

12. Elliot C. Cutler and S. A. Levine, "Cardiotomy and Valvulotomy for Mitral Stenosis. Experimental Observations and Clinical Notes concerning an Operated Case with Recovery," *Boston Medical & Surgical Journal* 88 (1923): 1023.

13. For quote see Harris B. Shumacker Jr., *The Evolution of Cardiac Surgery* (Indianapolis: Indiana University Press, 1992), p. 40.

14. John C. Munro, "Ligation of Ductus Ateriosus," *Annals of Surgery* 46 (1907): 335.

15. Robert E. Gross and John P. Hubbard, "Surgical Ligation of a Patent Ductus Arteriosus. Report of First Successful Case" *Journal of the American Medical Journal* (1939): 112, 729.

16. Robert E. Gross and Charles A. Hufnagel, "Coarctation of the Aorta. Experimental Studies Regarding Its Surgical Correction," *New England Journal of Medicine* (1945): 233, 287.

17. Robert E. Gross, "Surgical Correction for Coarctation of the Aorta," *Surgery* 18 (1945): 673.

18. See Stephen Westaby, *Landmarks in Cardiac Surgery* (Oxford: ISIS Medical Media, 1997), p. 93.

19. Robert E. Gross, "Treatment of Certain Aortic Coarctations by Homologous Grafts: A Report of 19 Cases," *Annals of Surgery* 134 (1951): 753.

20. Alfred Blalock and Helen Taussig, "The Surgical Treatment of Malformations of the Heart in Which There Is Pulmonary Stenosis or Atresia," *Journal of the American Medical Association* 128 (1945): 189.

21. C. S. Beck, W. H. Pritchard, and S. Fell, "Ventricular Fibrillation Abolished by Electric Shock," *Journal of the American Medical Association* 135 (1947): 985.

22. Paul M. Zoll, "Resuscitation of the Heart in Ventricular Standstill by External Electrical Stimulation," *New England Journal of Medicine* 247 (1952): 768.

23. Stephen Westaby, *Landmarks in Cardiac Surgery*, p. 30.

24. William M. Chardack, Andrew M. Gage, and Wilson Greatbatch, "A Transistorized, Self-Contained, Implantable Pacemeaker for the Long-Term Correction of Complete Heart Block," *Surgery* 48 (1960): 643.

25. Adrian Kantrowitz et al., "The Treatment of Complete Heart Block with an Implantable, Controllable Pacemaker," *Surgery, Gynecology & Obstetrics* 115 (1961): 415.

26. M. Mirowski et al., "Termination of Malignant Ventricular Arrythmias with an Implanted Automatic Defibrillator in Human Beings," *New England Journal of Medicine* 303 (1980): 322.

27. W. C. Sealy, "The Wolff-Parkinson-White Syndrome and the Beginnings of Direct Arrythmia Surgery," *Annals of Thoracic Surgery* 38 (1984): 176.

28. James L. Cox, "Cardiac Surgery for Arrythmias," *Journal of Cardiovascular Electrophysiology* 15 (2004): 25.

29. Horace G. Smithy, John A. Bone, and J. Stallworth, "Surgical Treatment of Constrictive Valvular Disease of the Heart," *Surgery, Gynecology & Obstetrics* 90 (1950): 175.

30. Charles Philamore Bailey, "Surgical Treatment of Mitral Stenosis (Mitral Commissurotomy)," *Diseases of the Chest* 15 (1949): 377.

31. Dwight E. Harken et al., "The Surgical Treatment of Mitral Stenosis. I. Valvuloplasty," *New England Journal of Medicine* 239 (1948): 801.

32. Dwight E. Harken et al., "The Surgery of Mitral Stenosis. III Finger-Fracture Valvuloplasty," *Annals of Surgery* 134 (1951): 722.

33. C. P. Bailey et al., "The Surgical Treatment of Aortic Stenosis," *Journal of Thoracic Surgery* 31 (1956): 375.

34. Charles P. Bailey et al., "The Surgical Correction of Mitral Insufficiency by the Use of Pericardial Grafts," *Journal of Thoracic Surgery* 30 (1954): 687.

35. Charles A. Hufnagel et al., "The Surgical Correction of Aortic Regurgitation," *Surgery* 35 (1954): 673.

36. C. P. Bailey et al., "Congenital Interatrial Communications: Clinical and Surgical Considerations with a Description of a New Surgical Technic: Atrio-septopexy," *Annals of Internal Medicine* 37 (1952): 888.

37. Robert E. Gross et al., "Surgical Closure of Defects of the Interauricular Septum by the Atrial Well," *New England Journal of Medicine* 247 (1952): 455.

38. For the sequence of events in the use of hypothermia see Shumacker, *The Evolution of Cardiac Surgery*, pp. 220–42.

39. C. Walton Lillehei, "Controlled Cross Circulation for Direct Vision Intracardiac Surgery," *Postgraduate Medicine* 17 (1955): 388.

40. John H. Gibbon Jr., "The Development of the Heart-Lung Apparatus," *Review of Surgery* 27 (1970): 231.

41. Harris B. Shumacker Jr., *A Dream of the Heart* (Santa Barbara, CA: Fithian Press, 1999)

42. John W. Kirklin et al., "Intracardiac Surgery with the Aid of a Mechanical Pump-Oxygenator (Gibbon Type). Report of Eight Cases," *Proceedings of the Staff Meetings, Mayo Clinic* 30 (1955): 201.

43. Clarence Dennis et al., "Development of a Pump-Oxygenator to Replace the Heart and Lungs; an Apparatus Applicable to Human Patients, an Application in One Case," *Annals of Surgery* 134 (1951): 709.

44. C. Walton Lillehei et al., "Direct Vision Surgery in Man Using a Simple, Disposable Artificial Oxygenator," *Diseases of the Chest* 29 (1956): 1.

45. Nina S. Braunwald, Theodore Cooper, and Andrew G. Morrow, "Complete Replacement of the Mitral Valve. Successful Clinical Application of a Flexible Polyurethane Prosthesis," *Journal of Thoracic Cardiovascular Surgery* 40 (1960): 12.

46. Albert Starr and M. Lowell Edwards, "Mitral Replacement: The Shielded Ball Valve Prosthesis," *Journal of Thoracic Cardiovascular Surgery* 42 (1961): 673.

47. Charles P. Bailey, Angelo May, and William M. Lemmon, "Survival after Coronary Endarterectomy in Man," *Journal of the American Medical Association* 164 (1957): 641.

48. Jack A. Cannon, William P. Longmire Jr., and Albert A. Kattus, "Considerations of the Rationale and Technique of Coronary Endarterectomy for Angina Pectoris," *Surgery* 46 (1959): 197.

49. David C. Sabiston Jr., "Direct Surgical Management of Congenital and Acquired Lesions of the Coronary Circulation," *Progress in Cardiovascular Diseases* 6 (1963): 299.

50. Rene G. Favaloro, "Saphenous Ven Autograft Replacement of Severe Segmental Coronary Artery Occlusion," *Annals of Thoracic Surgery* 58 (1969): 178, and W. Dudley Johnson et al., "Extended Treatment of Severe Coronary Artery Disease: A Total Surgical Approach," *Annals of Surgery* 170 (1969): 460.

51. C. William Hall et al., "Intraventricular Artificial Heart," *American Society of Artificial Organ Transpantation* 11 (1963): 263

52. O. H. Frazier, "First Use of an Unthethered, Vented Electric Left Ventricular Assist Device for Long-term Support," *Circulation* 89 (1994): 2908.

53. W. C. DeVries, "The Permanent Artificial Heart: Four Case Reports," *Journal of the American Medical Association* 259 (1988): 849.

54. Williams S. Pierce, "The Artificial Heart," in *Surgery of the Chest*, eds. Davis C. Sabiston Jr. and Frank C. Spencer. (Philadelphia: William B. Saunders, 1990).

CHAPTER 11

1. Yuriy Y. Voronoy, "Sobre Bloqueo del Aparato Reticuloendotelial de Hombre en Algunas Formas de Intoxication por el Sublimado y sobre la Transplantacion del Rinon Cadaverico como Metodo de Tratamiento de la Anuria Consecutiva a Aquella Intoxicacion," *Siglo Medico* 97 (1937): 296.

2. R. H. Lawler et al., "Homotransplantation of the Kidney in the Human," *Journal of the American Medical Association* 144 (1950): 844.

3. See Carl G. Groth, "Landmarks in Clinical Renal Transplantation," *Surgery, Gynecology & Obstetrics* 134 (1972): 323.

4. T. Gibson and P. B. Medawar, "Fate of Skin Grafts in Man," *Journal of Anatomy* 77 (1942–1943): 299.

5. Leslie Brent, *A History of Transplantation Immunology* (London: Academic

Press, 1997), p. 72.

6. D. M. Hume et al., "Experiences with Renal Transplantation in the Human: Report of Nine Cases," *Journal of Clinical Investigation* 34 (1955): 327.

7. J. B. Brown, "Homografting of Skin; with Report of Success in Identical Twins," *Surgery* 1 (1957): 558.

8. Joseph E. Murray, *Surgery of the Soul* (Canton, MA: Science History Publications, 2001), p. 80.

9. J. E. Murray, J. P. Merrill, and J. H. Harrison, *Surgical Forum* 6 (1955): 432, and "Kidney Transplantation between Identical Twins," *Annals of Surgery* 148 (1958): 343.

10. Ron Shapiro, Richard L. Simmons, and Thomas E. Starzl, *Renal Transplantation* (Stamford, CT: Appleton & Lange, 1977), p. 29.

11. Ibid., table 2-1, p. 30.

12. T. E. Starzl, T. L. Marchioro, and W. R. Waddell, "The Reversal of Rejection in Human Renal Homografyts with Subsequent Development of Tolerance," *Surgery, Gynecology & Obstetrics* 124 (1963): 395.

13. I. L. Lichtenstein and R. M. Barshak, "Experimental Transplantation of the Pancreas in Dogs," *Jounral of the International College Surgeons* 28 (1957): 1.

14. K. Reemtsma et al., "Islet Cell Function of the Transplanted Canine Pancreas," *Annals of Surgery* 90 (1963): 645.

15. W. D. Kelly et al., "Allotransplantation of the Pancreas and Duodenum along with the Kidney in Diabetic Neuropathy," *Surgery* 61 (1967): 827.

16. R. C. Lillehei et al., "Transplantation of the Pancreas," *Acta Endocrinologica*, suppl. 205 (1976): 303.

17. M. L. Gliedman et al., "Clinical Segmental Pancreatic Transplantation with Ureter-Pancreatic Duct Anastomosis for Exocrine Drainage," *Surgery* 74 (1973): 171.

18. V. Tellis, F. J. Vieth, and M. L. Gliedman, "Ten-Year Experience with Human Pancreatic Transplantation," *Transplantation Proceedings* 12, 4 suppl. 2 (1980): 78.

19. H. W. Sollinger, K. Cook, and D. Kamps, "Clinical and Experimental Experience with Pancreaticocystostomy for Exocrine Pancreatic Drainage in Pancreas Transplantation," *Transplantation Proceedings* 16 (1984): 749.

20. T. E. Starzl et al., "Pancreaticoduodenal Transplantation in Humans," *Surgery, Gynecology & Obstetrics* 159 (1984): 265.

21. A. C. Gruessner and D. E. R. Suthererland, "Pancreas Transplant Outcomes for United States (US) and non-US Cases as Reported to the United Network for Organ Sharing (UNOS) and the International Pancreas Transplant Registry (IPTR) as of June 2004," *Clinical Transplantation* 19 (2005): 433.

22. P. E. Lacy and M. Kostianovsky, "Method for the Isolation of Intact Islets of Langerhans for the Rat Pancreas," *Diabetes* 16 (1967): 35.

23. R. Younozai, R. L. Sorenson, and A. W. Lindall, "Homotransplantation of Isolated Pancreatic Islet Cells," *Diabetes*, suppl. (1970): 406.

24. W. F. Ballinger and P. E. Lacy, "Transplantation of Intact Pancreatic Islets in Rats," *Surgery* 72 (1972): 175.

25. J. S. Najarian et al., "Human Islet Transplantation: A Preliminary Report," *Transplantation Proceedings* 9 (1977): 233.

26. A. G. Tzakis et al., "Pancreatic Islet Cell Transplantation after Upper Abdominal Exentration and Liver Replacement," *Lancet* 336 (1990): 402.

27. D. E. R. Sutherland and R. W. G. Gruessner, "History of Pancreas Transplantation," in *Transplantation of the Pancreas*, ed. D. E. R. Sutherland and W. R. G. Gruessner (New York: Spinger-Verlag, 2004).

28. A. M. J. Shapiro et al., "Transplantation in Seven Patients with Type 1 Diabetes Mellitus Using a Glucocorticoid-Free Immunosuppressive Regimen," *New England Journal of Medicine* 343 (2000): 230.

29. T. E. Starzl with the assistance of C. W. Putnam, *Experiences in Hepatic Transplantation* (Philadelphia: W. B. Saunders, 1969), p. 349, fig. 158.

30. T. E. Starzl and H. W. Magoun, "Organization of the Diffuse Thalamic Projection System," *Journal of Neurophysiology* 14 (1951): 133.

31. C. S. Welch, "A Note on the Transplantation of the Whole Liver in Dogs," *Transplant Bulletin* 2 (1955): 54.

32. K. B. Absolon et al., "Experimental and Clinical Heterotopic Liver Homotransplantation," *Revue internationale d'hépatologie* 15 (1965): 1481.

33. F. D. Moore et al., "Experimental Whole Organ Transplantation of the Liver and Spleen," *Annals of Surgery* 152 (1960): 374.

34. T. E. Starzl and H. A. Haup Jr., "Mass Homotransplantation of Abdominal Organs in Dogs," *Surgical Forum* 11 (1960): 28.

35. T. E. Starzl et al., "Homotransplantation of the Liver in Humans," *Surgery, Gynecology & Obstetrics* 117 (1963): 659.

36. T. E. Starzl et al., "Orthotopic Homotransplantation of the Human Liver," *Annals of Surgery* 168 (1968): 392.

37. T. E. Starzl, *The Puzzle People* (Pittsburgh: University of Pittsburgh Press, 1992).

38. S. Todo et al., "Cadaveric Small Bowel and Small Bowel-Liver Transplantation in Humans," *Transplantation* 53 (1992): 369.

39. T. E. Starzl et al., "Heart-Liver Transplantation in a Patient with Familial Hypercholesterolemia," *Lancet* 1 (1984): 1382.

40. Sir Francis Darwin, *Eugenics Review* 6 (1914): 1.

41. F. C. Mann et al., "Transplantation of the Intact Mammalian Heart," *Archives of Surgery* 26 (1933): 219.

42. See Harris B. Shumacker Jr., *The Evolution of Cardiac Surgery* (Indianapolis: University of Indiana Press, 1992).

43. W. R. Webb and H. S. Howard, "Restoration of Function of the Refrigerated Heart," *Surgical Forum* 8 (1953): 302, and W. R. Webb et al., "Heart Preservation and Transplantation. Experimental and Clinical Studies," *American Journal of Cardiology* 22 (1968): 820.

44. R. R. Lower et al., "Successful Homotransplantation of the Canine Heart after Preservation for Seven Hours," *American Journal of Surgery* 104 (1962): 302.

45. N. E. Shumway and R. R. Lower, "Special Problems in Transplantation of the Heart," *Annals of the New York Academy of Sciences* 170 (1965): 773.

46. J. D. Hardy et al., "Heart Transplantation in Man. Report of the Initial Case," *Journal of the American Medical Association* 188 (1964): 1132.

47. J. D. Hardy et al., "Lung Transplantation in Man. Report of the Initial Case," *Journal of the American Medical Association* 186 (1963): 1065.

48. C. N. Barnard, "A Human Cardiac Transplant: An Interim Report of a Successful Operation Performed at Groote Schuur Hospital, Cape Town, South Africa," *South African Medical Journal* 41 (1967): 1271.

49. A. Kantrowitz et al., "Transplantation of the Heart in an Infant and an Adult," *American Journal of Cardiology* 22 (1968): 782.

50. D. A. Cooley et al., "Organ Transplantation for Advanced Cardiopulmonary Disease," *Annals of Thoracic Surgery* 8 (1969): 30.

51. C. F. Heck, S. J. Shumway, and M. P. Kaye, "The Registry of the International Society of Heart Transplantation: Sixth Official Report—1989," *Journal of Heart Transplantation* 8 (1990).

52. B. A. Reitz et al., "Heart-Lung Transplantation. Successful Therapy for Patients with Pulmonary Vascular Disease," *New England Journal of Medicine* 306 (1982): 557.

53. "2006 Annual Report of the US Organ Procurement and Transplantation Network and the Scientific Registry of Transplant Recipients. Transplant Data 1996–2005." Health Resources and Service Administration, Healthcare Systems Bureau, Division of Transplantation, Rockville, MD.

Chapter 12

1. J. O. Roe, "The Correction of Nasal Deformities," *Laryngoscopy* 18 (1908): 782.

2. Chevelier Jackson, *The Life of Chevalier Jackson, an Autobiography* (New York: Macmillan, 1938).

3. Hayes Elmer Martin, *Surgery of Head and Neck Tumors* (New York: Hoeber-Harper, 1964).

4. M. S. Strong and J. Jako, "Laser Surgery in the Larynx: Early Clinical Experience with Continuous CO2 Laser," *Annals of Otology, Rhinology, and Laryngology* 81 (1972): 791.

5. W. F. House, "Surgical Exposure of the Internal Auditory Canal and Its Contents through the Middle Cranial Fossa," *Laryngoscopy* 71 (1961): 1363.

6. G. Buck, "An Improved Method of Treating Fractures of the Femur," *Bulletin of the New York Academy of Medicine* 2 (1857): 233.

7. B. E. Hadra, "Wiring the Spinous Processes in Pott's Disease," *Medical Times and Register* 22 (1891): 413.

8. R. A. Hibbs, "An Operation for Progressive Spinal deformities," *Bulletin of the New York Academy of Medicine* 93 (1911): 1013.

9. P. R. Harrington, "The History and Development of Harrington Instrumentation," *Clinical Orthopaedics* 93 (1973): 110.

10. D. B. Phemister, "Operative Arrestment of Longitudinal Growth of Bones in the Treatment of Deformities," *Journal of Bone and Joint Surgery* 64 (1937): 287.

11. W. P. Blount and G. R. Clarke, "Control of Bone Growth by Epiphyseal Stapling," *Journal of Bone and Joint Surgery* (1949): 464.

12. M. R. Smith-Peterson, "Treatment of Fractures of the Neck of the Femur by Internal Fixation," *Surgery, Gynecology & Obstetrics* 64 (1937): 287.

13. H. H. Young, "Conservative Perineal Prostatectomy; Presentation of New Instruments and Technique," *Journal of the American Medical Association* 41 (1903): 999; H. H. Young, "The Early Diagnosis and Radical Cure of Carcinoma of the Prostate," *Bulletin of the Johns Hopkins Hospital* 16 (1905): 315.

14. P. C. Walsh, H. Lepor, and J. C. Eggleston, "Radical Prostatectomy with Preservation of Sexual Function: Anatomical and Pathological Considerations," *Prostate* 4 (1983): 473.

15. E. M. Bricker, "Bladder Substitution after Pelvic Eviseration," *Surgical Clinics of North America* 30 (1950): 1511.

16. W. E. Dandy, "Ventriculography following the Injection of Air into the Cerebral Ventricle," *Annals of Surgery* 68 (1918): 5; W. E. Dandy, "Roentgenography of the Brain after the Injection of Air into the Spinal Canal," *Annals of Surgery* 70 (1919): 397.

17. W. E. Dandy, "Intracranial Aneurysm of the Internal Carotid Artery. Cured by Operation," *Annals of Surgery* 107 (1938): 654.

18. W. E. Dandy, "Intracranial Hydrocephalus, an Experimental, Clinical, and Pathological Study," *American Journal of Diseases of Children* 8 (1914): 406.

19. W. E. Dandy, "The Diagnosis and Treatment of Hydrocephalus Resulting from Strictures of the Aqueduct of Sylvius," *Surgery, Gynecology, and Obstetrics* 31 (1920): 340.

20. See I. J. Wallman, "Shunting for Hydrocephalus: an Oral History," *Neurosurgery* 11 (1982): 308.

21. J. E. Goldthwaite, "The Lumbosacral Articulation. An Explanation of Many Causes of 'Lumbago,' 'Sciatica,' and Paraplegia," *Boston Medical and Surgical Journal* 164 (1911): 365.

22. W. J. Mixter and J. S. Barr, "Rupture of the Intervertebral Disc with Involvement of the Spinal Canal," *New England Journal of Medicine* 211 (1934): 210.

23. E. T. Ely, "An Operation for Prominence of the Ears," *Archives of Otolaryngology* 10 (1881): 97.

24. W. H. Luckett, "A New Operation for Prominent Ears Based on the Anatomy of the Deformity," *Surgery, Gynecology & Obstetrics* 10 (1910): 635.

25. T. L. Gilmer, "A Case of Fracture of the Lower Jaw with Remarks of the Treatment," *Archives of Dentistry* 4 (1887): 388–90.

26. V. P. Blair, "Underdeveloped Lower Jaw, with Limited Excursion," *Journal of the American Medical Association* 53 (1909): 178.

27. W. E. Ladd, "Surgical Diseases of the Alimentary Tract in Children," *New England Journal of Medicine* 216 (1936): 705.

28. W. E. Ladd, "The Surgical Treatment of Esophageal Atresia and Tracheoesophageal Fistula," *New England Journal Medicine* 230 (1944): 265; N. L. Leven, "Congenital Atresia of the Esophagus with Tracheoesophageal Fistula," *Journal of Thoracic Surgery* 10 (1941): 648.

29. C. Haight, "Congenital Atresia of the Esophagus with Tracheoesophageal Fistula. Reconstruction of Esophageal Continuity by Primary Anastomosis," *Annals of Surgery* 120 (1944): 62.

30. O. Swenson, E. B. D. Neuhauser, and L. K. Pickett, "New Concepts of Etiology, Diagnosis and Treatment of Hirschsprung's Disease," *Pediatrics* 4 (1949): 201.

31. P. L. Gliuck et al., "Correction of Congenital Hydronephrosis in Utero. IV. In Utero Decompression Prevents Renal Dysplasia," *Jounral of Pediatric Surgery* 19 (1984): 649; M. R. Harrison et al., "Correction of Congenital Diaphragmatic Hernia In Utero VII. A Prospective Trial," *Journal Pediatric Surgery* 32 (1997): 1637.

Chapter 13

1. Harvey Cushing, letter to Dr. Henry Christian, November 20, 1911.

2. L. K. Diamond, "A History of Blood Transfusion," in *Blood, Pure and Eloquent*, ed. M. M. Wintrobe (New York: McGraw-Hill, 1980).

3. G. W. Crile, *Hemorrhage and Transfusion* (New York: D. Appleton, 1909).

4. Ibid., p. 413.

5. Ibid., p. 533.

6. R. Lewisohn, "Blood Transfusion by the Citrate Method," *Surgery, Gynecology & Obstetrics* 21 (1915): 37.

7. R. Lewisohn, "The Frequency of Gastrojejunal Ulcers," *Surgery, Gynecology & Obstetrics* 40 (1925): 70.

8. C. E. Huggins, "Frozen Blood," *Journal of the American Medical Association* 193 (1965): 941.

9. J. H. Gibbon, "Post-operative Treatment," *Annals of Surgery* 46 (1907): 298.

10. W. G. Penfield and D. Teplitsky, "Prolonged Intravenous Infusion and the Clinical Determination of Venous Pressure," *Archives of Surgery* 7 (1923): 111.

11. R. Matas, "The Continued Intravenous Drip," *Annals of Surgery* 79 (1924): 643.

12. J. L. Gamble, *Chemical Anatomy, Physiology and Pathology of Extracellular Fluid* (Cambridge, MA: Harvard University Press, 1947).

13. For early history of fluid and electrolyte therapy see L. R. Mengoli, "Excerpts from the History of Postoperative Fluid Therapy," *American Journal of Surgery* 121 (1971): 311.

14. H. T. Randall, "Water and Electrolyte Balance in Surgery," *Surgical Clinics of North America* 32 (1952): 445.

15. G. T. Shires, "Shock and Metabolism," *Surgery, Gynecology & Obstetrics* 124 (1967): 284.

16. F. P. Underhill et al., "Blood Concentration Changes in Extensive Superficial Burns, and their Significance for Systemic Treatment," *Archives of Internal Medicine* 12 (1923): 31.

17. O. Cope and F. D. Moore, "The Redistribution of Body Water and the Fluid Therapy of the Burned Patient," *Annals of Surgery* 126 (1947): 1010.

18. E. I. Evans, "The Early Management of the Severely Burned Patient," *Surgery, Gynecology & Obstetrics* 94 (1952): 273.

19. E. Reiss et al., "Fluid and Electrolytes Balance in Burns," *Journal of the American Medical Association* 152 (1953): 1309.

20. C. R. Baxter and G. T. Shires, "Physiological Response to Crystalloid Resuscitation of Severe Burns," *Annals of the New York Academy of Sciences* 150 (1968): 874.

21. O. Cope et al., "Expeditious Care of Full Thickness Burn Wounds by Surgical Excision and Grafting," *Annals of Surgery* 125 (1947): 1.

22. J. C. Tanner et al., "The Mesh Skin Graft," *Plastic and Reconstructive Surgery* 34 (1964): 287.

23. J. F. Burke et al., "Successful Use of a Physiologically Viable Artificial Skin in the Treatment of Extensive Burn Injury," *Annals of Surgery* 194 (1981): 413.

24. S.T. Boyce et al., "Comparative Assessment of Cultured Skin Substitutes and Native Skin Autograft for Treatment of Full-Thickness Burns," *Annals of Surgery* 222 (1995): 743.

25. F. D. Moore, *Metabolic Care of the Surgical Patient* (Philadelphia and London: W. B. Saunders, 1959).

26. S. J. Dudrick et al., "Long-Term Parenteral Nutrition with Growth, Development, and Positive Nitrogen Balance," *Surgery* 64 (1968): 134.

27. R. H. Bartlett, "Extracorporeal Life Support: History and New Directions," *ASAIO Journal* 51 (2005): 487.

28. J. Folkman, "Tumor Angiogenesis: Therapeutic Implications," *New England Journal of Medicine* 285 (1971): 1182.

29. J. Folkman, "Is Angiogenesis an Organizing Principle in Biology and Medicine?" *Journal of Pediatric Surgery* 42 (2007): 1.

BIBLIOGRAPHY

General

Rutkow, Ira M. *American Surgery: An Illustrated History*. Philadelphia: Lippincott-Raven, 1998.

Preface

Absolom, Karel B. *The Surgeon's Surgeon: Theodor Billroth 1829–1890*. Lawrence, KS: Coronado Press, 1981.

Chapter 1: Pre-Columbian and Colonial Times

Breasted, James Henry. *The Edwin Smith Surgical Papyrus, Published in Facsimile and Hieroglyphics Transliteration with Translation and Commentary.* Chicago: University of Chicago Press, 1930.

Bulletin no. 34. Washington, DC: Government Printing Office, 1908.

Catesby, Mark. *The Natural History of Carolina, Florida, and the Bahama Islands.* London: C. Marsh, 1754.

Earle, A. Scott, ed. *Surgery in America: From the Colonial Era to the Twentieth Century.* 2nd ed. New York: Praeger Publishers, 1983.

Favata, Martin A., and Jóse B. Fernández. *The Account: Álvar Núñez Cabeza de Vaca's Relación.* Houston: Arte Público Press, 1993.

Hrdli ka, Aleš. *Physiological and Medical Observations among the Indians of Southwestern United States and Northern Mexico*. Washington, DC: Bureau of American Ethnology, 1900.

Lawson, John. *History of North Carolina*. Richmond, VA: Garrett & Massie, 1937.

Peltier, Leonard F. "John Jones: An Extraordinary Surgeon." *Surgery* 59 (1966): 633.

Thwaites, Reuben Gold. *John Long's Journal, 1768–1782*, vol. 2, *Early Western Travels, 1748–1846*. Cleveland: Arthur H. Clark, 1904.

Vogel, Virgil J. *American Indian Medicine*. Norman: University of Oklahoma Press, 1970.

CHAPTER 2: THE PROFESSOR AND THE PIONEER

American National Biography, vol. 17. New York: Oxford University Press, 1999.

Bell, John. "Philip Syng Physick." In *American Medical Biography: Lives of Eminent Physicians and Surgeons of the Nineteenth Century*, edited by Samuel D. Gross. Philadelphia: Lindsay and Blakiston, 1861.

Earle, A. Scott, ed. *Surgery in America*. 2nd ed. New York: Praeger, 1983.

Gross, Samuel D. *Memorial Oration in Honor of Ephraim McDowell.* Louisville, KY: John P. Morton, 1879.

Henderson, Thomas. "Correspondence." *Eclectic Repertory and Analytical Review* 8 (1818).

Johnson, James. "Editorial." *Medico-Chirugical Review* (January 1825–October 1826).

Lizars, John. "Observations on Extirpation of the Ovaria, with Cases."*Edinburgh Medical Journal* 12 (1824).

McDowell, Ephraim. "Observations of Diseased Ovaria." *Eclectic Repertory and Analytical Review* 9 (1819).

———. "Three Cases of Extirpation of Diseased Ovaria." *Eclectic Repertory and Analytical Review* 8 (1817).

Michener, Ezra. "Correspondence." *Eclectic and Analytical Review* 8 (1818).

Schachner, August. *Ephraim McDowell "Father of Ovariotomy" and Founder of Abdominal Surgery.* Philadelphia: J. B. Lippincott, 1921.

CHAPTER 3:THE BEGINNING OF CLINICAL EXPERIMENTATION— BIRTH OF A SPECIALTY

Beaumont, William. *Experiments and Observations on the Gastric Juice and the Physiology of Digestion.* Plattsburgh, NY: F. P. Allen, 1833.

———. "Further Experiments with the Case of Alexis St. Martin, Who Was Wounded in the Stomach by a Load of Duck-Shot, Detailed in the *Recorder* for Jan. 1, 1825." *Medical Recorder of Original Papers and Intelligence in Medicine and Surgery* 7 (1825): 94.

Combe, Andrew. *Experiments and Observations on the Gastric Juice and the Physiology of Digestion, by William Beaumont, M. D. of the United States Army.* Reprinted with notes. Edinburgh: 1838.

Lovell, Joseph. "A Case of Wounded Stomach by Joseph Lovell, Surgeon General, U.S.A." *Medical Recorder of Original Papers and Intelligence in Medicine and Surgery* 8 (1825): 14.

Myer, Jesse S. *Life and Letters of William Beaumont.* St. Louis: C. V. Mosby, 1912.

Chapter 4: Focus on Females

Alexson, D. E. "Women as Victims of Medical Experimentation: J. Marion Sims's Surgery on Slave Women 1845–1850." *Sage: A Scholarly Journal on Black Women* 2 (1985).

American National Biography, vol. 20. New York: Oxford University Press, 1999.

Barker-Benfield, G. J. *The Horrors of the Half-Known Life.* New York: Harper & Row, 1976.

Harris, Seale. *Woman's Surgeon: The Life Story of J. Marion Sims.* New York: Macmillan, 1950.

Kaiser, Irwin H. "Reappraisals of J. Marion Sims." *American Journal of Obstetrics & Gynecology* 132 (1978): 878–84.

Sims, J. Marion. *Clinical Notes on Uterine Surgery, with Special Reference to the Management of the Sterile Condition.* New York: W. Wood, 1866.

———. "The Discovery of Anesthesia." *Virginia Medical Monthly* 4 (1877): 81.

———. "Operation for Double Congenital Harelip." *American Journal of Dental Science* 5 (1844): 51.

———. *The Story of My Life.* New York: D. Appelton, 1888.

———. "Treatment of Vesico-Vaginal Fistula." *American Journal of Medical Science* 23 (1852): 59.

Chapter 5: The Death of Pain

Bigelow, H. J. "Insensibility during Surgical Operations Produced by Inhalation." *Boston Medical and Surgical Journal* 35 (1846): 309–17.

Boland, Frank Kells. *The First Anesthetic: The Story of Crawford Long.* Athens: University of Georgia Press, 1950.

Davy, Humphry. *Researches, Chemical and Philosophical, Chiefly concerning Nitrous Oxide.* London: J. Johnson, 1800.

Duncum, Barbara M. *The Development of Inhalation Anaesthesia.* London: Oxford University Press, 1947.

Fülöp-Miller, René. *Triumph over Pain.* New York: Literary Guild of America, 1938.

Hickman, H. *Letter on Suspended Animation, Containing Experiments Showing That It May Be Safely Employed during Operations on Animals, with the View of Ascertaining Its Probable Utility in Surgical Operations on the Human Subject.* Ironbridge: W. Smith, 1824.

Keys, T. E. *History of Surgical Anesthesia.* New York: Schuman, 1945.

Long, C. W. "An Account of the First Use of Sulphuric Ether by Inhalation as an

Anaesthetic in Surgical Operations." *Southern Medical and Surgical Journal* 5 (1849).

Mitchell, S. Weir. *The Complete Poems of S. Weir Mitchell.* New York: Century, 1914.

Sims, J. Marion. "Discovery of Anesthesia." *Virginia Medical Monthly* 4 (1877): 81.

Warren, J. C. *Etherization with Surgical Remarks.* Boston: W. D. Ticknor, 1848.

———. "Inhalation of Ether Vapor for the Prevention of Pain in Surgical Operations." *Boston Medical & Surgical Journal* 35 (1846): 375.

Young, Hugh H. "Long, the Discoverer of Anesthesia: A Presentation of the Original Documents." *Johns Hopkins Hospital Bulletin* 8 (1897): 174.

CHAPTER 6: TWO PRIME TARGETS

Gallbladder

Bobbs, John Stough. "Case of Lithotomy of the Gall-Bladder." *Transactions of the Indiana State Medical Society* 18 (1868): 68.

Brayton, Alembert W. "Dr. John S. Bobbs of Indianapolis, the Father of Cholecystotomy—His Original Paper on Lithotomy of the Gall Bladder." *Indiana Medical Journal* 18 (1899–1900): 177.

Kempner, G. W. H. "Affections of the Gall-Bladder Tending to Result in Cutaneous Biliary Fistula." *Transactions of the Indiana State Medical Society* 29 (1879): 120.

Sims, J. Marion. "Cholecystostomy in Dropsy of the Gall-Bladder." *British Journal of Medicine* 1 (1878): 811.

Sparkman, Robert S. "Bobbs Centennial: The First Cholecystostomy." *Surgery* 61 (1967): 873.

———. "Dr. John S. Bobbs of Indiana, the First Cholecystotomist."*Journal of Indiana State Medical Association* 60 (1967): 541.

———. "Mary Wiggins Burnsworth of Indiana, the First Person to Undergo Operation upon the Gallbladder." *Journal of Indiana State Medical Association* 1 (1967): 1.

Tait, Lawson. "Cholecystotomy for Dropsy of the Gall-Bladder due to Impaction of Gall-Stone." *Lancet* 2 (1879): 729.

Appendix

Fitz, Reginald H. "Perforating Inflammation of the Vermiform Appendix with Special Reference to Its Early Diagnosis and Treatment." *American Journal of Medical Science* 92 (1886): 108.

Fowler, George R. *A Treatise on Appendicitis*. Philadelphia: J. B. Lippincott, 1894.

Grant, W. W. "The Medical and Surgical History of the Vermiform Appendix." *Colorado Medicine* 30 (1933): 280.

Groves, A. *All in a Day's Work: Leaves from a Doctor's Notebook.* Toronto: Macmillan, 1934.

Herrington, J. Lynwood. "The Vermiform Appendix: Its Surgical History." *Contemporary Surgery* 39 (1991): 36.

Murphy, John B. "Two-Thousand Operations for Appendicitis and Deductions from His Personal Experience." *American Journal of Medical Science* 125 (1904): 187.

Ochsner, A. J. *Handbook of Appendicitis*. Chicago: G. P. Engelhard, 1906.

Chapter 7: Two Oft-Forgotten Contributions

John Shaw Billings

Chesney, Alan M. *The Johns Hopkins Hospital and the Johns Hopkins University School of Medicine*, vol. 1. Baltimore: Johns Hopkins Press, 1943.

Garrison, Fielding H. *John Shaw Billings: A Memoir.* New York: G. P. Putnam's Sons, 1915.

Lydenberg, Harry Miller. *John Shaw Billings.* Chicago: American Library Association, 1924.

———. *Selected Papers of John Shaw Billings*. Medical Library Association, 1965.

William Stuart Halsted

Cameron, John L. "William Stewart Halsted." *Annals of Surgery* 225 (1997): 445.

Halsted, W. S. "Refusion in the Treatment of Carbonic Oxide Poisoning." *New York Medical Journal* 38 (1883): 625.

MacCallum, W. G. *Surgical Papers by William Stewart Halsted 1852–1922*. Baltimore: Johns Hopkins Press, 1924.

———. *William Stewart Halsted, Surgeon.* Baltimore: Johns Hopkins Press, 1930.

CHAPTER 8: PRODIGY AND PROGENITOR

Bailey, Percival, and Harvey Cushing. *A Classification of the Tumors of the Glioma Group on a Histogenetic Basis with a Correlated Study of Prognosis*. Philadelphia: J. B. Lippincott, 1926.

Bliss, Michael. *Harvey Cushing: A Life in Surgery*. New York: Oxford University Press, 2005.

Codman, E. A. "Report of Results in Nontraumatic Surgery of the Brain and Spinal Cord. Observations on the Actual Results of Cerebral Surgery at the Massachusetts General Hospital." *Boston Medical and Surgical Journal* 153 (1905): 74.

Cushing, Harvey W. *A Bio-bibliography of Andreas Vesalius*. New York: Schuman, 1943.

———. "Concerning the Poisonous Effect of Pure Sodium Chloride Solutions on the Nerve-Muscle Preparations." *American Journal of Physiology* 6 (1901): 77.

———. "Electro-surgery as an Aid to the Removal of Intracranial Tumors. With a Preliminary Note on a New Surgical-current Generator by W. T. Bovie, PhD, Chicago." *Surgery, Gynecology & Obstetrics* 47 (1928): 751.

———. *From a Surgeon's Journal 1915–1918*. Boston: Little, Brown, 1936.

———. "Hematomyelia from Gunshot Wounds." *American Journal of Medical Science* 145 (1898): 654.

———. "The Hypophysis Cerebri: Clinical Aspects of Hyperpituitarism and Hypopituitarism." *Journal of the American Medical Association* 21 (1910): 127.

———. "Instruction in Operative Medicine, with the Description of a Course in the Hunterian Laboratory of Experimental Medicine." *Johns Hopkins Hospital Bulettin* 17 (1908): 124.

———. *Intracranial Tumors: Notes upon a Series of Two Thousand Verified Cases with Surgical Mortalities Pertaining Thereto*. Springfield, IL: Charles C. Thomas, 1932.

———. *Life of Sir William Osler*. New York and London: Oxford Press, 1925.

———. *Meningiomas*. Springfield, IL: Charles C. Thomas, 1932.

———. "A Method of Total Extirpation of the Gasserian Ganglion for Trigeminal Neuralgia. By a Route through the Temporal Fossa and beneath the Middle Meningeal Artery." *Journal of the American Medical Association* 34 (1900): 1035.

———. *The Pituitary Body and Its Disorders*. Philadelphia: J. B. Lippincott, 1912.

———. "The Sensory Distribution of the Fifth Cranial Nerve." *Johns Hopkins Hospital Bulletin* 15 (1904): 213.

———. "The Special Field of Neurological Surgery—Five Years Later." *Johns Hopkins Hospital Bulletin* 21 (1910): 325.

———. *Tumors of the Nervus Acusticus and the Syndrome of the Cerebellopontine Angle*. Philadelphia: W. B. Saunders, 1917.

CHAPTER 9: VICTORY OVER VESSELS

Barker, W. F., and J. A. Cannon. "An Evaluation of Endarterectomy." *Archives of Surgery* 66 (1955): 488.

Blaisdell. F. W., and A. D. Hall. "Axillo-Femoral Bypass for Lower Extremity Ischemia." *Surgery* 54 (1963): 563.

Carrea, R., M. Mollins, and G. Murphy. "Surgical Treatment of Spontaneous Thrombosis of the Internal Carotid Artery in the Neck. Carotid-Carotideal Anastomosis. Report of a Case." *Acta Neurologica Latiniomericana* 1 (1955): 71.

Carrel, A. "Anastomose bout a bout de la Jugulaire et de la Carotide Primitive." *Lyon Médical* 99 (1902): 114.

———. "La technique opératoire des anastomosis vasculaires et la transplantation des viscères." *Lyon Médical* 98 (1902): 859.

Cohen, Isidore, and Herman B. Deutsch. *Rudolph Matas*. Garden City, NY: Doubleday, 1960.

DeBakey, M. E., E. Stanley Crawford, George C. Morris Jr., and Denton A. Cooley. "Surgical Considerations of Occlusive Disease of the Innominate, Carotid, Subclavian, and Vertebral Arteries." *Annals of Surgery* 154 (1961): 698.

DeBakey, M. E., and F. A. Simeone. "Battle Injuries of the Arteries in World War II." *Annals of Surgery* 123 (1946): 534.

Dörfler, J. "Uber Arterieunaht." *Beitrag Zur Klinischen Chirurgie* 25 (1899): 781.

Dotter, C. T. "Transluminally-Placed Coil Spring Endarterial Tube Grafts. Long-Term Patency in Canine Popliteal Artery." *Investigative Radiology* 4 (1969): 329.

Eastcott, H. H. G., G. W. Pickering, and C. Rob. "Reconstruction of the Internal Carotid Artery in a Patient with Intermittent Attacks of Hemiplegia." *Lancet* 2 (1954): 994.

Edwards, W. Sterling, and Peter D. Edwards. *Alexis Carrel Visionary Surgeon.* Springfield, IL: Charles C. Thomas, 1974.

Fogarty, T. J., et al. "A Method of Extraction of Arterial Emboli and Thrombi." *Surgery, Gynecology & Obstetrics* 116 (1963): 241.

Freeman, N. E., et al. "Thromboendarterectomy for Hypertension due to Renal Artery Occlusion." *Journal of the American Medical Association* 156 (1954): 1077.

Friedman, Steven G. *A History of Vascular Surgery.* 2nd ed. Malden, MA: Blackwell Futura, 2005.

Garrison, Fielding H. *An Introduction to the History of Medicine.* 4th ed. Philadelphia: W. B. Saunders, 1929.

Greenfield, L. J., et al. "A New Intracaval Filter Permitting Continual Flow and Resolution of Emboli." *Surgery* 73 (1973): 599.

Gross, R. E., A. Bill, and E. C. Pierce II. "Methods for Preservation and Transplantation of Arterial Grafts. Observations on Arterial Grafts in Dogs, Report of Transplantation of Preserved Arterial Grafts in 9 Human Cases." *Surgery, Gynecology & Obstetrics* 88 (1949): 689.

Homans, J. "The Operative Treatment of Varicose Veins and Ulcers Based upon a Classification of These Lesions." *Surgery, Gynecology & Obstetrics* 22 (1916): 43.

———. "Thrombosis of the Deep Veins of the Lower Leg Causing Pulmonary Embolism." *New England Journal of Medicine* 211 (1934): 993.

Hufnagel, C. A. "Preserved Homologous Arterial Transplants." *Bulletin for the American College of Surgeons* 32 (1947): 231.

Hughes, C. W. "Acute Vascular Trauma in Korean War Casualties: An Analysis of 180 Cases." *Surgery, Gynecology & Obstetrics* 99 (1954): 91.

Jacobson, J. H., and E. L. Suarez. "Microsurgery in the Anastomosis of Small Vessels." *Surgical Forum* 11 (1968): 243.

Jahnke, E. J., Jr., and J. M. Howard. "Primary Repair of Major Arterial Injuries." *Archives of Surgery* 66 (1953): 646.

Kistner, R. "Surgical Repair of a Venous Valve." *Straub Clinical Procedures* 34 (1968): 41.

Lindbergh, Charles A. "An Apparatus for the Culture of Whole Organs." *Journal of Experimental Medicine* 62 (1935): 409.

Linton, R. R. "The Communicating Veins of the Lower Leg and the Operative Technic for their Ligation." *Annals of Surgery* 107 (1938): 582.

Malinin, Theodore I. *Surgery and Life: The Extraordinary Career of Alexis Carrel.* New York: Harcourt Brace Jovanovich, 1979.

Matas, R. "An Operation for the Radical Cure of Aneurysm Based on Arteriorraphy." *Annals of Surgery* 37 (1903): 16.

———. "Personal Experiences in Vascular Surgery: A Statistical Synopsis." *Annals of Surgery* 112 (1940): 802.

———. "Traumatic Aneurysm of the Left Brachial Artery." *Medical News Philadelphia* (1888): 462.

Moore, Wesley S. *Vascular and Endovascular Surgery.* 7th ed.Philadelphia: Saunders Elsevier, 2006.

Murphy, J. B. "Resection of Arteries and Veins Injured in Continuity-End-to-End Suture: Experimental and Clinical Research." *Medical Record* 51 (1897): 73.

Parodi, J. C., J. C. Palmaz, and H. D. Barone. "Transfemoral Intraluminal Graft Implantation for Abdominal Aortic Aneurysms." *Annals of Vascular Surgery* 5 (1991): 491.

Rutkow, Ira M. "Valentine Mott (1785–1865), the Father of American Vascular Surgery: A Historical Perspective." *Surgery* 85 (1979): 441.

Shaw, R. S., and R. H. Rutledge. "Superior-Mesenteric-Artery Embolectomy in Treatment of Massive Mesenteric Ischemia." *New England Journal of Medicine* 257 (1957): 595.

Spencer, F. C. "Plication of the Inferior Vena Cava." *Surgery* 62 (1967): 388.

Spencer, F. C., and R. V. Grewe. "The Management of Arterial Injuries in Battle Casualties." *Annals of Surgery* 141 (1955): 304.

Strully, K. J., E. S. Hurwitt, and H. W. Blankenberg. "Thromboendarterectomy for Thrombosis of the Internal Carotid Artery in the Neck." *Journal of Neurosurgery* 10 (1953): 474.

Voorhees, Arthur B., Jr., Alfred Jaretzki, and Arthur H. Blakemore. "The Use of Tubes Constructed from Vinyon 'N' Cloth in Bridging Arterial Defects." *Annals of Surgery* 135 (1952): 332.

Whipple, A. O. "The Problem of Portal Hypertension in Relation to the Hepatosplenopathies." *Annals of Surgery* 122 (1945): 449.

Chapter 10: Besting the Chest

Bailey, Charles P. "Surgical Treatment of Mitral Stenosis (Mitral Commissurotomy)." *Diseases of the Chest* 15 (1949): 377.

Bailey, Charles P., Angelo May, and William M. Lemmon. "Survival after Cardiac Endarterectomy in Man." *Journal of the American Medical Association* 164 (1957): 641.

Bailey, Charles P., et al. "Atrio-septo-pexy for Interauricular Septal Defects." *Journal of Thoracic Surgery* 26 (1953): 184.

Bailey, Charles P., et al. "The Surgical Correction of Mitral Insufficiency by the Use of Pericardial Grafts." *Journal of Thoracic Surgery* 30 (1954): 687.

Bailey, Charles P., et al. "The Surgical Treatment of Aortic Stenosis." *Journal of Thoracic Surgery* 31 (1956): 375.

Beck, C. S., W. H. Pritchard, and H. S. Feil. "Ventricular Fibrillation of Long Duration Abolished by Electric Shock." *Journal of the American Medical Association* 351 (1947): 985.

Bigelow, W. G., W. K. Lindsay, and W. F. Greenwood, "Hypothermia: Its Possible Role in Cardiac Surgery." *Annals of Surgery* 133 (1950): 830.

Blalock, Alfred, et al. "The Treatment of Myasthenia Gravis by Removal of the Thymus Gland." *Journal of the American Medical Association* 117 (1941): 1529.

Blalock, A., and H. B. Taussig. "The Surgical Treatment of Malformations of the Heart in Which There Is Pulmonary Stenosis or Pulmonary Atresia." *Journal of the American Medical Association* 128 (1945): 189.

Braunwald, Nina S., Theodore Cooper, and Andrew G. Morrow. "Complete Replacement of the Mitral Valve: Successful Clinical Application of a Flexible Polyurethane Prosthesis." *Journal of Thoracic Cardiovascular Surgery* 40 (1960): 12.

Brock, R. C. "Pulmonary Valvulotomy for Relief of Congenital Pulmonary Stenosis." *British Medical Journal* 1 (1948): 1121.

Callaghan, J. C., and W. G. Bigelow. "An Electrical Artificial Pacemaker for Standstill of the Heart." *Annals of Surgery* 134 (1951): 8.

Chardack, William M., Andrew A. Gage, and Wilson Greatbatch. "A Transistorized, Self-Contained Implantable Pacemaker for the Long-Term Correction of Complete Heart Block." *Surgery* 48 (1960): 643.

Cooley, Denton A., et al. "Orthotopic Cardiac Prosthesis for Two-Staged Cardiac Replacement." *American Journal of Cardiology* 24 (1969): 723.

Cooley, Denton A., et al. "Total Artificial Heart in Two-Staged Cardiac Transplantation." *Texas Heart Institute Journal* 8 (1981): 305.

Cox, James, L. "Cardiac Surgery for Arrythmias." *Journal of Cardiovascular Electrophysiology* 15 (2004): 25.

Cutler, E. C., and S. A. Levine. "Cardiotomy and Valvulotomy for Mitral Stenosis. Experimental Observations and Clinical Notes concerning an Operated Case with Recovery." *Boston Medical & Surgery Journal* 188 (1923): 1023.

Dalton, H. C. "Report of a Case of Stab-Wound of the Pericardium, Terminating in Recovery after Resection of a Rib and Suture of the Pericardium." *Annals of Surgery* 21 (1895): 147.

DeBakey, Michael E. "Left Ventricular Bypass Pump for Cardiac Assistance." *American Journal of Cardiology* 27 (1971): 3.

Dennis, Clarence, et al. "Development of a Pump Oxygenator to Replace the Heart and Lungs: An Apparatus Applicable to Human Patients, and Application to One Case." *Annals of Surgery* 134 (1951): 709.

DeVries, W. C. "The Permanent Artificial Heart. Four Case Reports." *Journal of the American Medical Association* 259 (1988): 849.

Favaloro, Rene G. "Saphenous Vein Autograft Replacement of Severe Coronary Artery Occlusion." *Annals of Thoracic Surgery* 5 (1968): 334.

Frazier, O. H. "First Use of an Untethered, Vented Electric Left Ventricular Assist Device for Long-Term Support." *Circulation* 89 (1994): 2908.

Garcelon, J. C., and J. P. O'Leary. "Dr. Rudolph Nissen: The Man and His Other Contributions." *American Journal of Surgery* 61 (1995): 468.

Graham, Evarts A. "Successful Removal of an Entire Lung for Carcinoma of the Bronchus." *Journal of the American Medical Association* 101 (1933): 1971.

Gross, Robert E. "Surgical Correction for Coarctation of the Aorta." *Surgery* 18 (1945): 673.

Gross, Robert E., and John P. Hubbard. "Successful Ligation of a Patent Ductus Arteriosus." *Journal of the American Medical Association* 112 (1939): 729.

Gross, Robert E., and Charles A. Hufnagel. "Coarctation of the Aorta, Experimental Studies Regarding its Surgical Correction." *New England Journal of Medical* 233 (1945): 287.

Gross, Robert E., et al. "Surgical Closure of Defects of the Interauricular Septum by Use of an Atrial Well." *New England Journal of Medicine* 247 (1951): 455.

Hall, C. W., et al. "Development of Artificial Intrathoracic Circulatory Pumps." *American Journal of Surgery* 108 (1964): 685.

Harken, Dwight E., et al. "Partial and Complete Prostheses in Aortic Insufficiency." *Journal of Thoracic Cardiovascular Surgery* 40 (1960): 744.

Harken, Dwight E., et al. "The Surgical Treatment of Mitral Insufficiency." *Journal of Thoracic Surgery* 28 (1954): 604.

Harken, Dwight E., et al. "The Surgical Treatment of Mitral Stenosis: Valvuloplasty." *New England Journal of Medicine* 239 (1948): 801.

Hill, L. I. "A Report of a Case of Successful Suturing of the Heart and Table of Thirty-seven Other Cases of Suturing by Different Operators with Various Terminations, and the Conclusions Drawn." *Medical Record* 62 (1902): 846.

Hufnagel, Charles A., et al. "The Surgical Correction of Aortic Regurgitation." *Surgery* 35 (1954): 673.

Johnson, Dudley W., et al. "Extended Treatment of Severe Coronary Artery Disease: A Total Surgical Approach." *Annals of Surgery* 170 (1969): 460.

Johnson, Stephen J. *The History of Cardiac Surgery: 1896–1955.* Baltimore: Johns Hopkins Press, 1970.

Kantrowitz, Adrian, et al. "The Treatment of Complete Heart Block with an Implantable, Controllable Pacemaker." *Surgery, Gynecology & Obstetrics* 115 (1961): 415.

Kirklin, John W., et al. "Intrathoracic Surgery with the Aid ofMechanical Pump Oxygenator System (Gibbon Type). Report of Eight Cases." *Clinical Proceedings of the Staff Meetings at the Mayo Clinic* 30 (1955): 105.

Kusserow, B. K. "A Permanently Indwelling Intracorporeal Pump to Substitute for Cardiac Function." *Transactions of the American Society for Artificial Internal Organs* 4 (1958): 227.

Lewis, F. John, and Mansur Taufic. "Closure of Atrial Septal Defects with the Aid of Hypothermia. Experimental Observations and the Report of One Successful Case." *Surgery* 33 (1953): 52.

Lilienthal, Howard. "Resection of the Lung for Supportive Infections with a Report Based on 31 Operative Cases in Which Resection Was Done or Intended." *Annals of Surgery* 75 (1922): 257.

Lillehei, C. W., et al. "The Results of Direct Vision Closure of Ventricular Septal

Defects in Eight Patients by Means of Controlled Cross Circulation." *Surgery, Gynecology & Obstetrics* 101 (1955): 447.

Longmire, William P., Jr., Jack A. Cannon, and Albert A. Kattus. "Direct-Vision Coronary Endarterectomy for Angina Pectoris." *New England Journal of Medicine* 259 (1958): 993.

Meltzer, S. J., and J. Auer. "Continuous Respiration without Respiratory Movements." *Journal of Experimental Medicine* (1909): 11.

Mirowski, M., et al. "Termination of Malignant Ventricular Arrhythmias with an Implanted Automatic Defibrillator in Human Beings." *New England Journal of Medicine* 303 (1980): 322.

Munro, John C. "Ligation of the Ductus Arteriosus." *Annals of Surgery* 46 (1907): 335.

Nissen, R. "Exstirpation eines ganzen Lungenfleugels." *Zentralblatt fur Chirurgie* 47 (1931): 303.

Norman, J. C., et al. "An Intracorporeal (Abdominal) Left Ventricular Assist Device: Initial Clinical Trials." *Archives of Surgery* 112 (1977): 142.

Norman, J. C., et al. "Total Support of the Circulation of a Patient with Post-cardiotomy Stone-Heart Syndrome by a Partial Artificial Heart (ALAVD) for 5 Days Followed by Heart and Kidney Transplantation." *Lancet* 1 (1978): 1125.

Pierce, William S. "The Artificial Heart." In *Surgery of the Chest*, 5th ed., edited by David C. Sabiston and Frank C. Spencer. Philadelphia: W. B. Saunders, 1990.

Ravitch, Mark M., ed. *The Papers of Alfred Blalock*. Baltimore: Johns Hopkins Press, 1966.

Richardson, Robert G. *The Surgeon's Heart*. London: William Heinemann Medical Books, 1969.

Romaine-Davis, Ada. *John Gibbon and His Heart-Lung Machine*. Philadelphia: University of Pennsylvania Press, 1991.

Sabiston, David C., Jr. "Direct Surgical Management of Congenital and Acquired Lesions of the Coronary Circulation." *Progress in Cardiovascular Disease* 6 (1963): 299.

Sealy, W. C. "The Wolff-Parkinson-White Syndrome and the Beginnings of Direct Arrhythmia Surgery." *Annals of Thoracic Surgery* 38 (1984): 176.

Sellors, T. Holmes. "Surgery of Pulmonary Stenosis: A Case in Which the Pulmonary Valve Was Successfully Divided." *Lancet* 1 (1948): 988.

Shumacker, Harris B., Jr. *The Evolution of Cardiac Surgery*. Bloomington: Indiana University Press, 1992.

Smithy, Horace G., John A. Bone, and J. Manley Stallworth. "Surgical Treatment of Constrictive Valvular Disease of the Heart." *Surgery, Gynecology & Obstetrics* 90 (1950): 175.

Starr, Albert, and M. Lowell Edwards. "Mitral Replacement: The Shielded Ball Valve Prosthesis." *Journal of Thoracic and Cardiovascular Surgery* 42 (1961): 673.

Torek, Franz. "The First Successful Case of Resection of the Thoracic Portion of the Oesophagus for Carcinoma." *Surgery, Gynecology & Obstetrics* 16 (1913): 614.

Varco, Richard. Discussion in William H. Muller and W. P. Longmire Jr. "The Surgical Treatment of Cardiac Valvular Stenosis." *Surgery* 30 (1951): 41.

Warden, Herbert E., et al. "Controlled Cross Circulation for Open Intracardiac Surgery." *Journal of Thoracic Surgery* 28 (1954): 331.

Westaby, Stephen, with Cecil Bosher. *Landmarks in Cardiac Surgery.* Oxford: Isis Medical Media, 1997.

Williams, Daniel H. "Stab Wound of the Heart and Pericardium—Recovery—Patient Alive Three Years Afterward." *Medical Record* 51 (1897): 437.

Zoll, Paul M. "Resuscitation of the Heart in Ventricular Standstill by External Electrical Stimulation." *New England Journal of Medicine* 247 (1952): 768.

Chapter 11: From One to Another—Organ Transplantation

Kidney

Brent, Leslie. *A History of Transplantation Immunology.* Oxford: Academic Press, 1997.

Brown, J. B. "Homografting of Skin: With Report of Success in Identical Twins." *Surgery* 1 (1937): 558.

Gibson, T. Medawar. "Fate of Skin Grafts in Man." *Journal of Anatomy* 77 (1942–1943): 299.

Groth, Carl G. "Landmarks in Clinical Renal Transplantation." *Surgery, Gynecology & Obstetrics* 134 (1972): 323.

Hume, D. H., et al. "Experiences with Renal Homotransplantation in the Human: Report of Nine Cases." *Journal of Clinical Investigation* 34 (1955): 327.

Lawler, R. H., J. W. West, P. H. McNulty, E. J. Clancy, and R. P. Murphy. "Homotransplantation of the Kidney in the Human." *Journal of the American Medical Association* 144 (1950): 844.

Merrill, J. P., et al. "Successful Transplantation from a Human Cadaver." *Journal of the American Medical Association* 185 (1963): 344.

Murray, Joseph E. *Surgery of the Soul.* Canton, MA: Science History Publications, 2001.

Murray, Joseph E., J. P. Merrill, and J. H. Harrison. "Kidney Transplantation between Seven Pairs of Identical Twins." *Annals of Surgery* 148 (1958): 343.

———. "Renal Homotransplantion in Identical Twins." *Surgical Forum* 6 (1955): 432.

Reemtsma, K., B. H. McCracken, and J. U. Schlegel. "Renal Heterotransplantation in Man." *Annals of Surgery* 160 (1964): 384–410.Shapiro, Ron, Richard L. Simmons, and Thomas E. Starzl. *Renal Transplantation.* Stamford, CT: Appleton & Lange, 1997.

Starzl, T. E., T. L. Marchioro, G. N. Peters, et al. "Renal Heterotransplantation from Baboon to Man: Experience with 6 Cases." *Transplantation* 2 (1964): 752–76.

Starzl, T. E., T. L. Marchioro, and W. R. Waddell. "The Reversal of Rejection in Human Renal Homografts with Subsequent Development of Tolerance." *Surgery, Gynecology & Obstetrics* 124 (1963): 395.

Voronoy, Yuriy Y. "Sobre bloque del aparato reticuloendotelial del hombre en algunas formas de intoxicacion por el sublimado y sobre la transplantacion del rinon cadaverico como metodo de tratamiento de la anuria consecutiva a aquella intocicacion." *El Siglo Medico* 97 (1937): 296.

Pancreas

Ballinger, Walter F., and Paul E. Lacy. "Transplantation of Intact Pancreatic Islets in Rats." *Surgery* 72 (1972): 175–86.

Gliedman, M. L., M. Gold, J. Whittaker, H. Rifkin, R. Sberman, S. Freed, V. Tellis, and F. J. Veith. "Clinical Segmental Pancreatic Transplantantion with Ureter-Pancreatic Duct Anastomosis for Exocrine Drainage." *Surgery* 74 (1973): 171–80.

Kelly, W. D., R. C. Lillehei, F. K. Merkel, Y. Idezuki, and F. C. Goetz. "Allotransplantation of the Pancreas and Duodenum along with the Kidney in Diabetic Nephropathy." *Surgery* 61 (1967): 827–35.

Lacy, P. E., and M. Kostianovsky. "Method for the Isolation of Intact Islets of Langerhans from the Rat Pancreas." *Diabetes* 16 (1967): 35.

Lichtenstein, I. L., and R. M. Barshak. "Experimental Transplantation of the Pancreas in Dogs." *Journal of the International College of Surgeons* 28 (1957): 1–6.

Lillehei, R. C., J. O. Ruiz, C. Aquino, and F. C. Goetz. "Transplantation of the Pancreas." *Acta Endocrinologica* 83 (1976): 303–20.

Najarian, J. S., D. R. Sutherland, M. W. Steffes, et al. "Human Islet Transplantation: A Preliminary Report." *Transplantation Proceedings* 9 (1977): 233–36.

Reemtsma, K., J. F. Lucas, R. E. Rogers, et al. "Islet Cell Function of the Transplanted Canine Pancreas." *Annals of Surgery* 90 (1963): 645–53.

Shapiro, A., J. Lakey, E. Ryan, et al. "Islet Transplantation in Seven Patients with Type 1 Diabetes Mellitus Using a Glucocorticoid-Free Immunosuppressive Regimen." *New England Journal of Medicine* 343 (2000): 230–38.

Sollinger, H. W., K. Cook, and D. Kamps. "Clinical and Experimental Experience with Pancreaticocystostomy for Exocrine Pancreatic Drainage in Pancreas Transplantation." *Transplantation Proceedings* 16 (1984): 749–51.

Starzl, T. E., S. Iwatsuki, B. W. Shaw Jr., D. A. Greene, D. H. Van Thiel, M. A. Nalesnik, J. Nuscbacher, H. Diliz-Pere, and T. R. Hakala. "Pancreaticoduodenal Transplantation in Humans." *Surgery, Gynecology & Obstetrics* 159 (1984): 265–72.

Sutherland, D., and R. Gruessner. "History of Pancreas Transplantation." In *Transplantation of the Pancreas*, edited by D. Sutherland and R. Gruessner. New York: Springer-Verlag, 2004.

———. "Pancreas Transplant Outcomes for United States (US) and non-US Cases as Reported to the United Network for Organ Sharing (UNOS) and the International Pancreas Transplant Registry (IPTR) as of June 2004." *Clinical Transplant* 19 (2005): 433–55.

Tellis, V., F. J. Veith, and M. L. Gliedman. "Ten Year Experience with Human Pancreatic Transplantation." *Transplantation Proceedings* 12 (1980) 78–80.

Tzakis, A. G., R. Ricordi, R. Alejandro, et al. "Pancreatic Islet Transplantation after Upper Aabdominal Exentration and Liver Replacement." *Lancet* 2 (1990): 402–405.

Younozai, R., R. L. Sorenson, and A. W. Lindall. "Homotransplantation of Isolated Pancreatic Islets." *Diabetes* 19 (1970): 406.

Liver

Absolon, K. B., P. F. Hagihara, W. O. Griffen Jr., and R. C. Lillehei. "Experimental and Clinical Heterotopic Liver Homotransplantation." *Revue internationale d'hépatologie* 15 (1965): 1481.

Moore, F. D., H. B. Wheeler, H. V. Demissianos, et al. "Experimental Whole-Organ Transplantation of the Liver and Spleen." *Annals of Surgery* 152 (1960): 374–87.

Starzl, T. E. *Experience in Hepatic Transplantation.* Philadelphia: W. B.Saunders, 1969.

———. *The Puzzle People.* Pittsburgh: University of Pittsburgh Press, 1992.

Starzl, T. E., et al. "Heart-Liver Transplantation in a Patient with Familial Hypercholesterolemia." *Lancet* 1 (1984): 1382.

Starzl, T. E., V. M. Bernhard, R. Benevuto, and N. Cortes. "A New Method for One-Staged Hepatectomy in Dogs." *Surgery* 46 (1959) 880–86.

Starzl, T. E., C. G. Groth, L. Brettschneider, et al. "Orthotopic Homotransplantation of the Human Liver." *Annals of Surgery* 168 (1968): 392–415.

Starzl, T. E., and H. A. Haupp Jr. "Mass Homotransplantation of Abdominal Organs in Dogs." *Surgical Forum* 11 (1960): 28–30.

Starzl, T. E., T. L. Marchioro, K. N. Van Kaulla, et al. "Homotranstplatation of the Liver in Humans." *Surgery, Gynecology & Obstetrics* 117 (1963): 659–76.

Starzl, T. E., S. Todo, M. Tzakis, et al. "The Many Faces of Multivisceral Organ Transplantation." *Surgery, Gynecology & Obstetrics* 172 (1991): 335–44.

Todo, S., A. G. Tzakis, K. Abu-Elmagd, et al. "Cadaveric Small Bowel and Small Bowel-Liver Transplantation in Humans." *Transplantation* 53 (1992): 369–76.

Welch, C. S. "A Note on Transplantation of the Whole Liver in Dogs." *Transplantation Bulletin* 2 (1955): 54.

Heart and Lung

Barnard, C. N. "A Human Cardiac Transplant: An Interim Report of Successful Operation Performed at Groote Schuur Hospital, Cape Town." *South Africa Medical Journal* (1967): 1271–74.

Carrel, Alexis. "The Surgery of Blood Vessels." *Johns Hopkins Hospital Bulletin* 18 (1907): 18–28.

Cooley, Denton A., Robert D. Bloodwell, Grady L. Hallman, James J. Nora, and Harrision M. Gunyon. "Organ Transplantation for Advanced Cardiopulmonary Disease." *Annals of Thoracic Surgery* 8 (1969): 30–46.

Hardy, James D., M. Carlos, Fred D. Kurrus, William A. Neely, et al. "Heart Transplantation in Man. Report of the Initial Case." *Journal of the American Medical Association* 188 (1964): 1132–40.

Hardy, James D., Watts R. Webb, Martin L. Dalton Jr., and George R. Walker Jr. "Lung Transplantation in Man. Report of the Initial Case." *Journal of the American Medical Association* 186 (1963): 1065–74.

Heck, Christopher F., Sara J. Shumway, and Micheal P. Kaye. "The Registry of the International Society of Heart Transplantation: Sixth Official Report—1989." *Journal of Heart Transplant* 8 (1990).

Kantrowitz, Adrian, Jordan D. Haller, Howard Joos, Narcial M. Derruti, and Hans E. Carstensen. "Transplantation of the Heart in an Infant and an Adult." *American Journal of Cardiology* 22 (1968): 782–90.

Lower, Richard, R., Raymond C. Stofer, Edward J. Hurley, Eugene Dong Jr., Roy B. Cohn, and Norman E. Shumway. "Successful Homotransplantation of the Canine Heart after Anoxic Preservation for Seven Hours." *American Journal of Surgery* 104 (1962): 302–306.

Mann, Frank C., James T. Priestly, J. Markowitz, and Wallace M. Yater. "Transplantation of the Intact Mammalian Heart." *Archives of Surgery* 26 (1933): 219–24.

Reitz, Bruce A., John Wallwork, Sharon A. Hunt, and Norman E. Shumway. "Heart-Lung Transplantation: Successful Therapy for Patients with Pulmonary Vascular Disease." *New England Journal of Medicine* 306 (1982): 557–74.

Shumacker, Harris B., Jr. *The Evolution of Cardiac Surgery*. Indianapolis: Indiana University Press, 1992.

Shumway, Norman E., and Richard R. Lower. "Special Problems in Transplantation of the Heart." *Annals of the New York Academy of Science* 170 (1965): 773–77.

Webb, Watts R., and Hector S. Howard. "Restoration of Function of the Refrigerated Heart." *Surgical Forum* 8 (1953): 302–306.

Webb, Watts R., Winfred L. Sugg, and Roger R. Ecker. "Heart Preservation and Transplantation. Experimental and Clinical Studies." *American Journal of Cardiology* 22 (1968): 820–25.

Westaby, Stephen, and Cecil Bosher. *Landmarks in Cardiac Surgery*. Oxford: Isis Medical Media, 1997.

Chapter 12: Smatterings from the Specialties

Otolaryngology

House, W. "Surgical Exposure of the Internal Auditory Canal and Its Contents through the Middle Cranial Fossa." *Laryngoscope* 71 (1961): 1363.

Jackson, Chevalier. *The Life of Chevalier Jackson: An Autobiography*. New York: Macmillan, 1938.

Martin, Hayes Elmer. *Surgery of Head and Neck Tumors*. New York: Hoeber-Harper, 1964.

Roe, J. O. "The Correction of Nasal Deformities." *Laryngoscope* 18 (1908): 782–97.

Strong, M. S., and G. J. Jako. "Laser Surgery in the Larynx: Early Clinical Experience with Continuous CO2 Laser." *Annals of Otology, Rhinology, and Laryngology* 81 (1972): 791.

Orthopaedics

Bick, Edgar M. *Classics of Orthopaedics*. Philadelphia: J. B. Lippincott, 1976.

Blount, Walter P., and George R. Clarke. "Control of Bone Growth by Epiphyseal Stapling." *Journal of Bone and Joint Surgery* 31–A (1949): 464–78.

Buck, G. "An Improved Method of Treating Fractures of the Femur Trans." *New York Academy of Medicine* 2 (1857): 233.

Bunnell, Sterling. *Surgery of the Hand.* Philadelphia: J. B. Lippincott, 1944.

Hadra, B. E. "Wiring the Spinous Processes in Pott's Disease." *Medical Times and Register* 22 (1891): 413.

Harrington, P. R. "The History and Development of Harrington Instrumentation." *Clinical Orthopaedics* 93 (1973): 110.

Hibbs, R. A. "An Operation for Progressive Spinal Deformities." *New York Medical Journal* 93 (1911): 1013.

Kanavel, Allan B. *Infections of the Hand.* Chicago: 1933.

LeVay, David. *The History of Orthopaedics.* Casterton Hall: Parthenon, 1990.

Phemister, D. B. "Operative Arrestment of Longitudinal Growth of Bones in the Treatment of Deformities." *Journal of Bone and Joint Surgery* 15 (1933): 1–15.

Smith-Peterson, Marius N. "Treatment of Fractures of the Neck of the Femur by Internal Fixation." *Surgery, Gynecology & Obstetrics* 64 (1937): 287.

Urology

Bricker, E. M. "Bladder Substitution after Pelvic Evisceration." *Surgical Clinics of North America* 30 (1950): 1511.

Young, H. H. "Conservative Perineal Prostatectomy: Presentation of New Instruments and Technique." *Journal of the American Medical Association* 41 (1903): 999.

———. "The Early Diagnosis and Radical Cure of Carcinoma of the Prostate." *Bulletin of the Johns Hopkins Hospital* 16 (1905): 315.

Walsh, P. C., H. Lepor, and J. C. Eggleston. "Radical Prostatectomy with Preservation of Sexual Function: Anatomical and Pathological Considerations." *Prostate* 4 (1983): 473.

Neurosurgery

Dandy, W. E. "The Diagnosis and Treatment of Hydrocephalus resulting from Strictures of the Aqueduct of Sylvius." *Surgery, Gynecology & Obstetrics* 31 (1920) 340–58.

———. "Intracranial Aneurysm of the Internal Carotid Artery. Cured by Operation." *Annals of Surgery* 107 (1938): 654–59.

———. "Roentgenography of the Brain after the Injection of Air into the Spinal Canal." *Annals of Surgery* 70 (1919): 397–403.

———. "Ventriculography following the Injection of Air into the Cerebral Ventricle." *Annals of Surgery* 68 (1981): 5–11.

Dandy, W. E., and K. D. Blackfan. "Internal Hydrocephalus, an Experimental, Clinical, and Pathological Study." *American Journal of Disease of Children* 8 (1914): 406–82.

Goldthwaite, J. E. "The Lumbosacral Articulation: An Explanation of Many Cases of 'Lumbago.'" *Boston Medical and Surgical Journal* 164 (1911): 365–72.

Greenblatt, Samuel H. ed. *A History of Neurosurgery: In Its Scientific and Professional Contexts.* Park Ridge, IL: American Association of Neurological Surgeons, 1997.

Mixter, W. J., and J. S. Barr. "Rupture of the Intervertebral Disc with Involvement of the Spinal Canal." *New England Journal of Medicine* 211 (1934): 210–15.

Wallman, I. J. "Shunting for Hydrocephalus: An Oral History." *Neurosurgery* 11 (1982): 308–13.

Plastic and Reconstructive Surgery

Blair, Vilray Papin. "Underdeveloped Lower Jaw, with Limited Excursion." *Journal of the American Medical Association* 53 (1909): 178.

Ely, Edward T. "An Operation for Prominence of the Auricles." *Archives of Otolaryngology* 10 (1881): 97.

Gilmer, Thomas L. "A Case of Fracture of the Lower Jaw with Remarks on the Treatment." *Archives of Dentistry* 4 (1887): 388–90.

Luckett, William H. "A New Operation for Prominent Ears Based on the Anatomy of the Deformity." *Surgery, Gynecology & Obstetrics* 10 (1910): 635–37.

McDowell, Frank. *The Source Book of Plastic Surgery.* Baltimore: Williams & Wilkins, 1977.

Pediatric Surgery

Glick, P. L., et al. "Correction of Hydronephrosis in Utero. IV: In Utero Decompression Prevents Renal Dysplasia." *Journal of Pediatric Surgery* 19: 649.

Haight, C. "Congenital Atresia of the Esophagus with Tracheoesophageal Fistula. Reconstruction of Esophageal Continuity by Primary Anastomosis." *Annals of Surgery* 120 (1944): 62.

Harrison, Michael R., et al. "Correction of Congenital Diaphragmatic Hernia in Utero. VII: A Prospective Trial." *Journal of Pediatric Surgery* 32 (1997): 1637.

Ladd, W. E. "Surgical Diseases of the Alimentary Tract in Children." *New England Journal of Medicine* 216 (1936): 705.

———. "The Surgical Treatment of Esophageal Atresia and Tracheoesophageal Fistula." *New England Journal of Medicine* 230 (1944): 265.

Leven, N. L. "Congenital Atresia of the Esophagus with Tracheoesophageal Fistula." *Journal of Thoracic Surgery* 10 (1941): 648.

Swenson, O., E. B. D. Neuhauser, and L. K. Pickett. "New Concepts of Etiology, Diagnosis and Treatment of Hirschsprung's Disease." *Pediatrics* 4 (1949): 201.

CHAPTER 13: ENABLING EXPANSION

Blood

Crile, George W. *Hemorrhage and Transfusion.* New York and London: D. Appleton, 1909.

Diamond, L. K. "A History of Blood Transfusion." In *Blood: Pure and Eloquent,* edited by Maxwell M. Wintrobe. New York: McGraw-Hill, 1980.

Huggins, C. E. "Frozen Blood." *Journal of the American Medical Association* 193 (1965): 941.

Lewisohn, R. "Blood Transfusion by the Citrate Method." *Surgery, Gynecology & Obstetrics* 21 (1915): 37.

———. "The Frequency of Gastrojejunal Ulcers." *Surgery, Gynecology & Obstetrics* 40 (1925): 70.

Fluid and Electrolytes

Gamble, James L. *Chemical Anatomy, Physiology and Pathology of Extracellular Fluid.* Cambridge, MA: Harvard University Press, 1947.

Gibbon, J. H. "Post-operative Treatment." *Annals of Surgery* 46 (1907): 298.

Matas, R. "The Continued Intravenous Drip." *Annals of Surgery* 79 (1924): 643.

Mengoli, Louis R. "Excerpts from the History of Postoperative Fluid Therapy." *American Journal of Surgery* 121 (1971): 311.

Penfield, W. G., and D. Teplitsky. "Prolonged Intravenous Infusion and the Clinical Determination of Venous Pressure." *Archives of Surgery* 7 (1923): 111.

Randall, Henry T. "Water and Electrolyte Balance in Surgery." *Surgical Clinics of North America* 32 (1952): 445.

Burns

Baxter, C. R., and G. T. Shires. "Physiological Response to Crystalloid Resuscitation of Severe Burns." *Annals of the New York Academy of Science* 150 (1969): 874.

Boswick, John A., Jr. *The Art and Science of Burn Care.* Rockville, MD: Aspen, 1987.

Boyce, S. T., et al. "Comparative Assessment of Cultured Skin Substitutes and Native Skin Autograft for Treatment of Full-Thickness Burns." *Annals of Surgery* 222 (1995): 742.

Burke, J. F., et al. "Successful Use of a Physiologically Viable Artificial Skin in the Treatment of Extensive Burn Injury." *Annals of Surgery* 194 (1981): 413.

Cope, O. "Expeditious Care of Full Thickness Burn Wounds by Surgical Excision and Grafting." *Annals of Surgery* 125 (1947): 1.
Cope, O., and F. D. Moore. "The Redistribution of Body Water and the Fluid Therapy of the Burn Patient." *Annals of Surgery* 126 (1947): 1010.
Evans, E. I. "The Early Management of the Severely Burned Patient." *Surgery, Gynecology & Obstetrics* 94 (1952): 273.
Herndon, David N. *Total Burn Care.* 3rd ed. Philadelphia: Saunders Elsevier, 2007.
Reiss, E., et al. "Fluid and Electrolyte Balance in Burns." *Journal of the American Medical Association* 152 (1953): 1309.
Shire, G. T. "Shock and Metabolism." *Surgery, Gynecology & Obstetrics* 124 (1967): 284.
Tanner, J. C., et al. "The Mesh Skin Graft." *Plastic and Reconstructive Surgery* 34 (1964): 297.
Underhill, F. P., et al. "Blood Concentration Changes in Extensive Superficial Burns, and Their Significance for Systemic Treatment." *Archives of Internal Medicine* 12 (1923): 31.

Metabolic Care of the Surgical Patient

Moore, Francis D. *Metabolic Care of the Surgical Patient.* Philadelphia and London: W. B. Saunders, 1959.

Nutritional Support

Dudrick, S. J., et al. "Long-Term Total Parenteral Nutrition with Growth, Development, and Positive Nitrogen Balance." *Surgery* 64 (1968): 134.

Extracorporeal Membrane Oxygenation (ECMO)

Bartlett, R. H. "Extracorporeal Life Support: History and New Directions." *American Society for Artificial Internal Organs Journal* 51 (2005): 487.

Anti-angiogenesis

Bliss, Michael. *Banting: A Biography.* Toronto: McClelland and Stewart, 1984.
Folkman, J. "Is Angiogenesis an Organizing Principle in Biology and Medicine?" *Journal of Pediatric Surgery* 42 (2007): 1.
———. "Tumor Angiogenesis: Therapeutic Implications." *New England Journal of Medicine* 285 (1971): 1182.

ILLUSTRATIONS

INDEX

Name Index

Locators in *italics* indicate illustrations.

SUBJECT INDEX

Locators in *italics* indicate illustrations.